MARY SEACOLE:
THE MAKING OF THE MYTH

MARY SEACOLE:
THE MAKING OF THE MYTH

LYNN MCDONALD

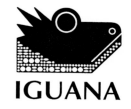

IGUANA

Published by Iguana Books
720 Bathurst Street, Suite 303
Toronto, Ontario, Canada
M5V 2R4

Publisher: Greg Ioannou
Editor: Kelly Lamb, Kathryn Willms
Front cover image and design: Ashley James
Book layout design: Meghan Behse

Library and Archives Canada Cataloguing in Publication

McDonald, Lynn, 1940-, author
        Mary Seacole : the making of the myth / Lynn McDonald.

Includes bibliographical references.
Issued in print and electronic formats.
ISBN 978-1-77180-055-6 (pbk.).--ISBN 978-1-77180-056-3 (epub).--ISBN 978-1-77180-057-0 (kindle).--ISBN 978-1-77180-058-7 (pdf)

        1. Seacole, Mary, 1805–1881. 2. Nurses--Jamaica--Biography. 3. Women, Black--Jamaica--Biography. 4. Crimean War, 1853–1856--Women--Jamaica. 5. Crimean War, 1853–1856--Medical care. I. Title.

RT37.S43M23 2014   610.73092   C2014-900867-8
                                             C2014-900868-6

This is an original print edition of *Mary Seacole: The Making of the Myth*.

To the memory of Dr John Sutherland

and the Sanitary Commission

unsung heroes of the Crimean War

Nightingale and Seacole
as portrayed at a soldier's bedside

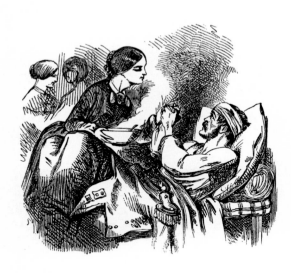

'The Nightingale's Song to the Soldier,' in *Punch* 4 November 1854, is a realistic portrayal of Nightingale, although the bed is far better than the straw pallets used for soldiers in the war hospitals. (Reproduced with permission of Punch Ltd., www.punch.co.uk)

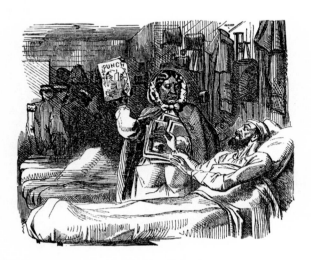

'Our Own Vivandière,' *Punch* 30 May 1857, shows Seacole as a hospital visitor giving a copy of *Punch* to a soldier (the stock soldier-in-hospital-bed image). Children's books frequently make Seacole into a nurse at the bedside (as shown on the cover and p x), in effect making Seacole into the Nightingale figure of the other cartoon. (Reproduced with permission of Punch Ltd., www.punch.co.uk)

Table of Contents

Dramatis Personae

Gleichen, Count (1833–91) Seacole customer and sculptor
Hall, John (Dr, Sir) (1815–66) principal medical officer
Herbert, Elizabeth (1822–1911) wife of secretary at war
Herbert, Sidney (1810–61) war secretary
Moore, Mary Clare (1814–74) superior, Sisters of Mercy, Bermondsey
Palmerston, Lord (1784–1865) prime minister
Panmure, Lord (1801–74) war secretary after Herbert
Raglan, Lord (1788–1855) commander of the British forces
Rokeby, Lord (1798–1883) Guards commander, chair of Seacole Fund
Smith, Andrew (Dr, Sir) (1797–1872) director, Army Medical Dept.
Soyer, Alexis (1809–58) volunteer chef for the British Army
Stratford de Redcliffe, Lord (1786–1880) British ambassador
Sutherland, John (Dr) (1808–91) head, Sanitary Commission

Other Authors/Eye Witnesses

Alexander, James Edward (Sir) (1803–85) regiment commander
Astley, John Dugdale (later Sir) (1828–94) Scots Fusilier Guards
Blackwood, Alicia (Lady) (1819–1913) wife of British chaplain
Blake, Ethelbert (Dr) (1818–97) regimental surgeon, 55th Foot Gds
Bracebridge, Charles H. (1799–1872) accompanied Nightingale nurses
Hamley, Edward Bruce (1824–93) aide-de-camp, military historian
Hamlin, Cyrus (1811–1900) American missionary, bread supplier
Keane, H. Fane (Hon) (1822–95) Royal Engineer, Seacole committee
Kinglake, A.W. (1809–91) war historian
MacDonald, J.C. (1822–89) *Times* Fund manager
Paget, George (Lord) (1818–80) commander, Light Brigade
Paulet, William (Lord) (1804–93) commandant of the Bosphorus
Porter, Whitworth (1827–92) officer, Royal Engineers
Reid, Douglas Arthur (Dr) (c1834–1924) British Army doctor
Roebuck, John Arthur (1801–79) MP, chair of Roebuck Committee
Russell, W.H. (later Sir) (1821–1907) *Times* war correspondent
Sabin, John Edward (1821–91) senior chaplain, British Army
Skene, James Henry (1812–86) diplomat in Turkey
Stafford, Augustus (1811–57) MP, witness at Roebuck Committee
Stanley, Mary (1813–79) leader of second nursing team
Tolstoy, Leo (1828–1910) Russian Artillery officer, novelist
Wood, Evelyn (1838–1919) Royal Navy, later field marshal

Seacole
portrayed as a nurse at a soldier's bedside

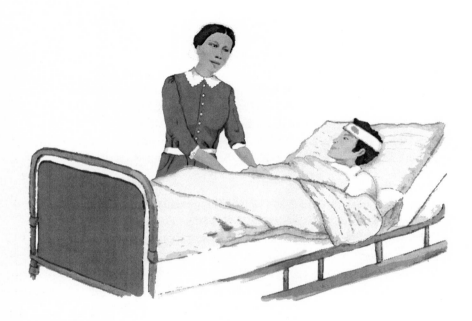

This portrayal of Seacole nursing at a soldier's bedside (also on the cover) is a composite of typical portrayals of her in children's books. Some show her as slim, some as heavier; nearly all dress her in a blue and white uniform, similar to what was worn (later) at the Nightingale School.

Preface

How is it that someone who never was a nurse, nor an expert on health care, should come to be promoted as the 'pioneer nurse' and to be named, by the UK Department of Health no less, a 'pioneer of health care' on a list on which Florence Nightingale is conspicuously absent? The person in question is Mary Seacole, a fine and decent woman, who never claimed to have been a nurse, nor to have contributed to health care reform in any way, while Nightingale was both the major founder of the modern profession of nursing and a visionary of quality health care for all — and successful in achieving many advances towards that high goal.

Both these women made their name in the Crimean War: Seacole as a Jamaican businesswoman running a store/restaurant/bar/takeaway/catering service for officers, with pro bono work as a 'doctress' or herbalist on the side; Nightingale as the leader of the first team of British women to nurse in war and whose research after the war documented what went wrong — the hospital death rates were appalling — with recommendations on how to ensure that such death rates would not recur.

The Department for Education decided in 2012 to drop Nightingale from the English National Curriculum, but to keep Seacole in, after rumours that she, too, would be dropped prompted a strong and successful campaign to save her. In 2013, after (more modest) interventions in favour of Nightingale, the department relented. At the present moment both women are represented on the English National Curriculum; however, the actual teaching on the two tends to exaggerate Seacole's contributions and detract from or ignore Nightingale's.

Nightingale's contributions are in danger of again being minimized by plans to erect a three-metre-tall bronze statue of Seacole at St Thomas'

Hospital, the home for more than a century of the Nightingale School and the base for decades of her pioneering work. Ironically, the statue is intended to face the Houses of Parliament, although Seacole never took up political causes, while Nightingale wrote briefs for Parliamentary committees, gave evidence to commissions and lobbied assiduously for improvements in health care, nursing and hospitals.

This powerful campaign to lionize Seacole at the expense of recognizing the contributions of Nightingale has been propagated by many national institutions as well as two government departments (Health and Education): the BBC, the National Army Museum, the National Portrait Gallery, the Royal Mail, the Royal College of Nursing, National Health Service Employers and trusts, nursing unions and university health care faculties.

I had never heard of Seacole when I began work on *The Collected Works of Florence Nightingale*, a sixteen-volume series published 2001–12. Yet she is now routinely given credit for Nightingale's work. News to me! As it would have been to Seacole, who left a fascinating memoir which contains only favourable accounts of Nightingale and no claims of comparable achievements.

Neither the adulation of Seacole nor the denigration of Nightingale can be accounted for by new historical discoveries. Numerous primary sources are available on both. A massive amount of information can be found on Nightingale and substantial enough material on Seacole for judgments to be made. What real primary sources say, including Seacole herself, will show how far the falsification project has gone.

This refiguring of history has also affected Nightingale's legacy in recent decades. For example, her brief, friendly encounter with Seacole has been distorted into a racist attack, by the BBC no less. As in other books, articles and online sources, anyone who deals with Seacole must also deal with Nightingale, especially now as the campaign proceeds to replace Nightingale with a new pioneer of nursing and health care. However, this book will focus on Seacole with references to Nightingale only where the two women crossed paths, as they did during the Crimean War, the only time they ever met.

Researching Seacole had its pleasures. The task was light compared with searching for and editing Nightingale's thousands of letters, books, articles and notes. Seacole left but one short book and several letters. She was an admirable person, generous, kind and good-humoured according to those who knew her. She is responsible only minimally for creating the misleading myths: she did wear medals never awarded her and the flattering testimonials she included in her book were likely fictional. However, she never claimed to have won any medals and even acknowledged in her memoir that she would have liked to. The memoir itself never promises a thorough or careful account, but 'wonderful adventures,' on which it delivers.

The falsification is recent, but it has spread so widely now that the most honest and diligent researcher would have difficulty getting the story right. Exaggerations and misstatements appear even in respectable print sources, although they are more frequent in websites and social media. Typically sources relay multiple myths or false statements, ranging from minor factual errors to far-fetched accusations. Seacole's engaging memoir serves often to expose the errors, giving an account quite at variance with what her supporters claim today. My research turned up much new material on Seacole, but nothing that would substantiate the claims of heroism or medals, and much to the contrary.

While responsibility for errors is mine alone, I would like to acknowledge much advice and assistance from colleagues: Patricia Warwick for website assistance and proofreading; Lesley Mann for census and other searches; Ken Simons for chart assistance; Wendy Mathews for documentation on the statue campaign; Tom Keighley for his considerable experience in the nursing profession; and to editors Kathryn Willms and Meghan Behse at Iguana Books. To them and to other colleagues who formed the Nightingale Society in 2012 to set the record straight, my thanks.

Lynn McDonald
Toronto
April 2014

Chapter 1

The myth of Mary Seacole: an introduction

Mary Seacole was a real person. She was born in Jamaican in 1805 (although she lied about her age in two UK censuses) and lived her retirement years in London, where she died in 1881. She led a remarkable life and left a fine memoir of her travels, *Wonderful Adventures of Mrs. Seacole in Many Lands*, published in 1857. Seacole grew up as a free, mixed-race Jamaican, three-quarters white, and lived largely in a white world (her husband was white, as were her business partner and clientele). Her mother ran an upmarket boarding house in a good location in Kingston, now the site of the Jamaican National Library. The family were prosperous, middle class and solidly pro-British in their sentiments. The boarding house catered largely to army and navy officers and their wives, contacts that would lead Seacole to the Crimean War of 1854–56.

Seacole and Florence Nightingale met at Nightingale's war hospital, near Constantinople, probably for only five minutes. They did not talk about nursing according to Seacole's memoir, the only source we have on this historic moment.[1] Nor would they have, for Seacole was not a nurse

---

[1] Mary Seacole, *Wonderful Adventures of Mrs Seacole in Many Lands* 89–90; all references to this work are to the 1988 Oxford edition, a facsimile edition with the same page numbers as the original.

and never claimed to be one; she called herself a 'doctress,' meaning a herbalist. She had tried to join the second group of nurses sent to the war but was not accepted (nothing to do with Nightingale) and when the two actually met Seacole was merely seeking a bed for the night, as she was on her way to meet her business partner in the Crimea to start their enterprise.

All this is quite different from the Mary Seacole of TV films, school and NHS websites, the popular media and even some serious books of history whose authors should know better. Seacole in such sources has become a nurse, even a 'black nurse' (she called herself 'yellow' to indicate her light complexion), and a war heroine with medals for bravery (although she never claimed any). How this mythologized Seacole came into being and how she came to be promoted as the replacement to Florence Nightingale are the main subjects of this book. In the course, the authentic Mary Seacole will emerge, what she did in the Crimean War, what Nightingale did and how the two related to each other.

Myth making

The boldest way of creating false history is for the perpetrator to write up fake documents, paying attention to the age of the paper, ink, etc., and insert them into the right file in an appropriate archive. Nothing in the creation of the Mary Seacole myth goes that far. Rather there has been an abundance of creative writing, crediting her with winning medals (from one to four) and inventing medal inscriptions (from mere bravery to 'bravery, kindness and saving lives'). Medal award ceremonies are conjured up, sometimes with Queen Victoria herself doing the honours. The myth makers have created first-person narratives for Seacole, complete with quotation marks. They've imaginatively erected whole hospitals, field hospitals, clinics, sick bays and nursing stations, when Seacole herself described only a humble hut for her store to serve customers and other huts for storage and living quarters for herself, her business partner and their employees. Her business, as she made clear, sold drinks, meals and takeaways to officers and catered for their social and sporting events, with a canteen for the soldiers. No matter! According to the mythologizers,

Seacole provided 'accommodation, food and nursing care' for ordinary soldiers, saving 'thousands of lives.'[2]

The myths have made their way onto artifacts, notably a plaque in the Mary Seacole Building at Brunel University with a picture showing her wearing three medals and calling her a 'pioneer nurse.' The Royal Mail helped to circulate the myths by putting her, again wearing those medals, on a postage stamp. Publicity for it ranked her as one of ten 'great Britons,' with six men (including Winston Churchill, William Shakespeare and Charles Darwin) and three other women (suffrage leader Emmeline Pankhurst, novelist Virginia Woolf and the founder of the hospice movement, Cicely Saunders). In 2013, she was further promoted to being one of four 'pioneers of health care,' with Edward Jenner (for smallpox vaccination), Elizabeth Garrett Anderson (the first woman medical dean) and Aneurin Bevan (who established the National Health Service in 1948) in whose names the Department of Health created awards for leadership. Nightingale is absent from both lists.

Florence Nightingale throughout has been a problem for Seacole supporters. Some acknowledge her sufficiently to claim kinship between them, such as the 'two nursing luminaries,'[3] or describing Seacole as the 'black Nightingale.' More often, however, Nightingale has been treated as an obstacle to be dealt with, and her legacy has been attacked with slurs on her work and a campaign of misinformation, although Seacole herself held no grudge against her, and the two, from the only records available from the time, spoke well of each other, as will be seen in Chapter 3.

That these myths have been so readily accepted testifies to the hold of today's political correctness and the effectiveness of indoctrination in the school system. Seacole and Nightingale have been taught together in the English National Curriculum since 2007, so that millions of people have

---

[2] Karen Sorenson, 'Mary Seacole Memorial Statue Update,' paper for Guy's and St Thomas' NHS Foundation Trust 20 July 2011.

[3] Elizabeth Anionwu, *A Short History of Mary Seacole: A Resource for Nurses and Students* 29.

learned that Seacole was the 'real,' 'hands-on' nurse and heroine[4] while Nightingale was a distant administrator, over rated as the 'lady of the lamp.' Political correctness is not necessarily a bad thing and certainly its motivation to redress historic discrimination is worthy. A basic requirement, however, is that it get the facts right.

A leaked government document in December 2012 revealed the intention to drop both Seacole and Nightingale from the English National Curriculum.[5] There was a great ruckus to keep Seacole in, beginning with a petition campaign by Operation Black Vote. Support for Nightingale to remain in the curriculum was restrained. In June 2013, the secretary of state for education announced that Nightingale would be dropped, but Seacole would remain. However, the department held a consultation on its draft new programme, to which the Nightingale Society, among other organizations, sent arguments for inclusion. In September 2013, the minister announced that the department had listened and would keep Nightingale on the curriculum.

Chapter 2 gives background on the Crimean War, now long distant, but notable for high death rates and interesting complications. Chapters 3 and 4 introduce the basic facts about Seacole and Nightingale, respectively, using documents from the time. Sources are all fully given, in sharp contrast with the practices of most of the Seacole myth makers.

Chapter 5 relates no less than ten myths or false statements about Seacole, again with full sources provided. For each of these statements there are multiple sources. They range from scholarly books by reputable academics, entries in well-known encyclopedias, and the websites of national institutions, such as the National Army Museum, the National Portrait Gallery, NHS trusts and the Department of Health itself. Each of the myths is refuted with data from the time, including Seacole's own

---

[4] National Portrait Gallery, 'Mary Seacole: Lost Portrait of Mary Seacole Discovered,' 10 January 2005; Sue Carpenter, 'The Forgotten Angel of the Crimea,' *The Times* 4 September 2000:12–13.

[5] 'Gove Faces War with Equality Activists as he Axes Labour's PC Curriculum that dropped Greatest Figures from History Lessons,' *Mail Online* 29 December 2012.

memoir, newspaper stories, and journal notes, letters and memoirs of participants in the Crimean War.

Chapter 6 gives excerpts from Seacole's *Wonderful Adventures*, which continues to delight and charm readers. Chapter 7 gives conclusions, such as they are, on what survives when the myths are debunked, with suggestions as to how Seacole and Nightingale might more realistically be taught and how better to recognize diversity in nursing.

A timeline at the end of this chapter sets out the life events for both Seacole and Nightingale to act as a reality checklist in considering their contributions to nursing and health care.

Top Black Briton

Mary Seacole was voted the top 'Black Briton' in 2004 and has assumed a status of role model in the UK, especially for nurses and other health care workers. Black Britons, and nurses of all ethnicities, will find much here that they will not have heard before. Some of it is negative, some decidedly positive, but much of it will challenge the popular myths surrounding Seacole.

Britons must ask themselves what kind of heroes and heroines they want and if falsifying history is acceptable. Seacole would hardly recognize herself in the statements now made about her by her overly enthusiastic admirers. Most of the myths are refutable from her own memoir, which it seems few of her supporters have ever read.

Nurses and health care workers might want to take another look at Nightingale, for she was the major founder of modern nursing, first set out the principles of environmental health and pioneered research on occupational health and safety for nurses. She worked for decades to make hospitals safer, advanced understanding of the social determinants of health (especially housing) and conducted the first British study of maternal mortality post-childbirth, all the while pressing for better working conditions and career opportunities for nurses. In 1864, she articulated the principles of public health care — even that the poor should get as good care as those better off. Nightingale not only made her mission the well-being of ordinary soldiers — as opposed to officers — she went on to examine the conditions that make for war and those that help to prevent it. It's time for a reappraisal of Nightingale, as well as a de-mythologizing of Seacole.

In the eye of the beholder

For some commentators, Nightingale even looks wrong, at least in comparison to Seacole. In her Introduction to a recent edition of *Wonderful Adventures*, the editor remarks on 'Nightingale's virginal pallor and purity,' compared with Seacole's 'robust maternity and patriotic spirit of enterprise.'[6] Mayor Boris Johnson's 2011 *Johnson's Life of London* has Nightingale looking 'down her beaky nose' at the vast numbers celebrating Mary Seacole at Surrey Gardens (Nightingale was not even there).[7] A review of a biography of Seacole describes Nightingale as 'pale and pinched.'[8] A Facebook entry is yet ruder, declaring that Nightingale 'looks like an uptight bitch in her photos.'[9]

A New Zealand Marxist nurse called Nightingale a 'nasty, small-minded, prissy piece of malevolence,' which you could see, she said, 'when you look at her picture...look at that pinched mouth. Look at those mean little eyes.' Seacole, by contrast, had a 'generous countenance, openness of mien and comfortable presentation.' Nightingale was further faulted for inventing the pie chart and starting 'this whole idea that nursing needs numbers.'[10]

---

[6] Sarah Salih, Introduction, *Wonderful Adventures of Mrs Seacole in Many Lands* xxxii.

[7] Boris Johnson, 'Florence Nightingale and Mary Seacole: Who pioneered nursing' 283.

[8] Kathryn Hughes, 'The Creole with the Teacup,' *Guardian* books 15 January 2005.

[9] 'Florence Nightingale World's Worst Nurse,' originally entitled 'Florence Nightingale was a Murdering Bitch,' 2012.

[10] Chris Cottingham, 'Signifying Mary: Move Over Florence — Nursing Has a New Mother. Well Guerilla Nursing That Is and It's Mrs Mary Seacole,' *Kai Tiaki: Nursing New Zealand* 17,5 (June 2011):5.

Of course none of these people actually saw Nightingale and those who did described her more favourably — although none as a great beauty — and she was pale and thin when recovering from her illness in the Crimea in 1855. Commenting on her shortly before she fell ill, the chef Alexis Soyer, who saw her almost daily for a year, described her 'physiognomy' as 'most pleasing':

> her eyes of a bluish tint speak volumes and are always sparkling with intelligence; her mouth is small and well formed....Her visage, as regards expression, is very remarkable and one can almost anticipate by her countenance what she is about to say...a gentle smile passes radiantly over her countenance;...at other times, when wit or a pleasantry prevails, the heroine is lost in the happy, good-natured smile which pervades her face.[11]

A chaplain who saw Nightingale frequently at the beginning of the war described her as having a manner and countenance that were 'prepossessing' but 'without the possession of positive beauty':

> It is a face not easily forgotten, pleasing in its smile, with an eye betokening great self-possession, and giving, when she wishes, a quiet look of firm determination to every feature. Her general demeanour is quiet and rather reserved.[12]

On meeting Nightingale back in London in 1856, a leading navy doctor commented: 'She has a most brilliant and intelligent smile, a very pleasant and not patronizing address.'[13]

Seacole was a middle-aged fifty when she arrived in the Crimea and was typically referred to as 'old.' Soyer's biographer called her a 'prodigiously fat and immensely good-natured old woman.'[14] Her portraits, busts and photographs all show her as a woman of mature years, but she is often

---

[11] Alexis Soyer, *Soyer's Culinary Campaign, Being Historical Reminiscences of the Late War* 153.

[12] S.G. Osborne, *Scutari and its Hospitals* 25.

[13] Richardson letter to his wife, 4 December 1856, John McIlraith, *The Life of Sir John Richardson* 251.

[14] Helen Morris, *Portrait of a Chef: The Life of Alexis Soyer* 165.

portrayed today as if in her twenties or thirties, ages more typical of the hospital nurse the myth makers want her to be. She took pride in her dress and hats and was always well turned out (she travelled with a maid). She favoured bright colours and ribbons, as will be seen in comments on her later.

Seacole used the colour 'yellow' to describe herself, indicating a fair complexion, as opposed to black. She never called herself black, but blacks appear in her memoir as employees, including her 'grinning black' barber (38) and 'good-for-nothing black cooks' (141). Yet she is regularly portrayed on book covers, Youtube and websites as young and black, often in a nurse's uniform complete with a modest white cap. Children's books, especially, depict her as a hospital nurse, decidedly young, slim and black.[15]

Myth making, falsifying, faking

Chapter 5 relates who said precisely what and when in the development of the Seacole myth. Two distinct themes can be identified, one pro-Seacole, the other anti-Nightingale, both dating to 1982.

The anti-Nightingale campaign effectively began with the publication of Australian historian F.B. Smith's *Florence Nightingale: Reputation and Power* in 1982. This book, which never mentions Seacole, denigrates Nightingale's work and character from its first page to its last. Then, in 1998, Hugh Small's *Florence Nightingale: Avenging Angel* attacks her Crimean War work, going so far as to blame her for the high death rates of the war hospitals — which she had exposed and worked to prevent recurring. (Refutations of both books are available.[16]) The few references to Seacole in

---

[15] Flagrant examples are Harriet Castor's *Mary Seacole* and Sylvia L. Collicott's *The Story of Mary Seacole*.

[16] Lynn McDonald, 'Florence Nightingale Revealed in her own Writings,' *The Literary Supplement* 6 December 2000:14–15; 'Appendix B: The Rise and Fall of Florence Nightingale's Reputation,' in Lynn McDonald, ed. *Florence Nightingale: Life and Family* 843–47; *Florence Nightingale at First Hand*; 'Florence Nightingale, Statistics and the Crimean War,' *Journal of the Royal Statistical Society* Series A online 7 October 2013.

that book show that Small fell for the core Seacole myths of medals and heroism. He then appeared in two major BBC films attacking Nightingale, and on one that was pro-Seacole, which also denounces Nightingale.

The Seacole campaign began with the publication of a short booklet, *Mary Seacole: Jamaican National Heroine and 'Doctress' in the Crimean War*, by Ziggi Alexander and Audrey Dewjee. It compares her favourably to Nightingale, crediting her with the 'skill of a surgeon,' 'healing hands' and a 'commitment to nursing,' adding the false accusation that she was rejected for a nursing post by Nightingale (2). It changes Seacole's account (in *Wonderful Adventures* 143) of providing coffee and breakfasts for officers to providing 'for off-duty soldiers' (11). There is no mention of serving champagne and catering for dinner parties or the elite visitors.

Then, in 1984, the same authors produced the first reissue of Seacole's *Wonderful Adventures of Mrs Seacole in Many Lands*, originally published in 1857. The reissue is welcome, for the book is still well worth a read, but the thirty-seven-page introduction[17] continued the misinformation of the booklet, claiming heroine status for Seacole, including the provision of 'excellent medical supervision' and the saving of 'many lives,' although it was cautious about the awarding of medals (35).

Also in 1984, the first endorsement of Seacole in a nursing journal appeared, in an editorial of the *Journal of Advanced Nursing*. It goes beyond the above sources in naming Seacole 'a black British nurse,' awarding her 'medical skills' and making a mild swipe at Nightingale.[18] In 1988, novelist Salman Rushdie entered the fray. In *The Satanic Verses*, he muses about characters of history: 'See, here is Mary Seacole, who did as much in the Crimea as another magic-lamping Lady, but, being dark, could scarce be seen for the flame of Florence's candle' (292). He had already ridiculed Nightingale, without mentioning Seacole, in his first novel *Grimus* where 'Mlle Florence Nightingale' is an obliging whore in a whorehouse (141).

---

[17] Ziggi Alexander and Audrey Dewjee, eds, Introduction 9–45.

[18] James P. Smith, 'Mary Jane Seacole 1805–1881: A Black British Nurse,' *Journal of Advanced Nursing* 9,5 (1984):427.

Rushdie's salute to Seacole in *The Satanic Verses* was subsequently plagiarized on a website of the National Army Museum (reference since removed). There the third-person account he gives becomes a first-person lament by Seacole: 'To the troops I was not the Lady with the Lamp. I, "being dark, could scarce be seen for the flame of Florence's candle." I was Mother Seacole.'

In 1991, Seacole was posthumously granted the Jamaican Order of Merit, the only medal that she actually won. On her being named the top 'Black Briton' in 2004, events moved rapidly, both in Jamaica and Britain. That year, Wolverhampton University became the first UK university to name a building after her, for its School of Health and Well-being. The year 2005 marked the 200th anniversary of her birth, which was celebrated in Jamaica by the placing of a historic plaque at her former boarding house and the issuing of four stamps in her honour. One shows pictures of four medals: the French Legion of Honour, the British Crimea, the Turkish Medjidie and the Jamaican Order of Merit, only the last of which she actually won.

The Mary Seacole stamp issued in 2006 was part of a series in honour of the 150th anniversary of the founding of the National Portrait Gallery in 1856. But 1856 is also notable as the end of the Crimean War and the beginning of Nightingale's lifelong work to establish nursing as a profession and to improve public health and hospitals. And while the founder of the hospice movement, Cicely Saunders (herself a Nightingale nurse), was one of the four women honoured, Nightingale was not. Incidentally, Nightingale's *Suggestions for Thought* influenced the writing of another honoree, Virginia Woolf, in her much-loved essay, 'A Room of One's Own.'

Also in 2006, no fewer than three British universities named buildings after Seacole, all variously praising her contributions as a leading nurse and heroine. Two of them display pictures of her with medals and the fraudulent claims.

The indoctrination of school children, from primary age up to the History GCSE, doubtless accounts for the high level of misinformation on Seacole (and Nightingale) in the general population. How widespread teaching on Seacole has been is not clear; inclusion in the National Curriculum does not require that the person be taught, nor omission forbid it. Websites and blogs by teachers show that correct answers are pro-Seacole and anti-Nightingale. A Youtube video made by children at Southwold Primary School, Hackney, for example, shows them demonstrating 'The A-Z of Mary Seacole,' complete with M for medals. At her Islington school, the daughter of Mayor Boris Johnson played Queen Victoria, pinning medals on both Seacole and Nightingale (283–84). The mayor knew that no such ceremony ever happened (305) so why did the school put it on?

An online source for preparation for GCSE history gives the 'best answer' to a question on the differences and similarities between Seacole and Nightingale as

> Seacole often tended wounded from both sides actually on the battlefield and under fire, which Nightingale never did. Nightingale and her nurses were officially recognized... [while] Seacole was strictly a volunteer.

This 'best answer' concludes that the two were 'equally important in improving medical care and treatment of injured soldiers,' and even in establishing 'the concept of modern nursing and its effectiveness' (posted 2011-06-14).

A good illustration of the misinformation conveyed in school sources can be seen in a lesson plan from Episode 9, 'The Life of Mary Seacole,' in BBC School Radio's 'History — The Victorians.'[19] The episodes and questions not only promote the new heroic portrayal of Seacole, but they seem designed to cause resentment against Nightingale. Which is the more effective pedagogical device, the use of leading questions or the provision of false answers?

> Key question: 'What obstacles did Mary Seacole overcome to serve as a nurse in the Crimean War?'

---

[19] This BBC School Radio lesson plan can be found at
http://downloads.bbc.co.uk/schoolradio/pdfs/history/mary_seacole.pdf

Instruction: 'Write down the things Mary Seacole overcame to fulfil her ambition.'

(Answers: Racism preventing travel to England from Jamaica. Not allowed to serve as a nurse in the army. Had to make the dangerous journey to the Crimea on her own.)

The website next poses a 'discussion question': 'What do soldiers need if they are injured fighting in a war?' The answer supplied is quite obvious: 'To be cleaned, bandaged, kept warm, brought food, given medicine,' none of which Seacole is known to have done.

The BBC lesson plan then goes on to a 'key question': 'How did Mary Seacole help the British soldiers?' and asks students to 'write notes to explain what Mary Seacole did to help the British soldiers.' Answers naturally follow that are not factual but repeat familiar myths: 'Providing shelter and food for injured soldiers. Running a hospital in a dangerous area close to where the battles took place.'

To foment resentment, the lesson plan explains that soldiers and Nightingale's nurses 'were all brought home by the British Army.' Seacole was not; the British Army did not supply transport to business people, for obvious reasons — not a point made on the website. The next 'discussion question' asks children to say how they think Seacole 'should have been treated after the Crimean War.'

BBC provides 'episode synopses' which cover important events in Seacole's life:

Her unsuccessful attempt to enlist as a nurse to help Florence Nightingale in the Crimean War leads to her decision to travel to the Crimea and set up her own hospital there; her courageous work on the battlefield tending to wounded soldiers; and finally, how she spent the years after the end of the war impoverished and unappreciated.

A new fiction appears that, after the war, back in London, Seacole was so poor that she could not keep on 'Sally, her faithful maid.' Sally, Seacole's first cheerleader, was 'angry that everyone seemed to have forgotten how much' she had done during the war. But if she did have a maid Sally, Seacole herself never mentioned her. Her maid in the Crimea, as in Panama, was a Mary (*Wonderful Adventures* 57) who probably did not return to London with her. (She is not mentioned again). A 'Sally' appears in Soyer's memoir as Seacole's daughter (269) but, again, she is never heard of again, and Soyer is the only source to mention her at all. Finally, the 'impoverished and unappreciated' point is also untrue. The trust fund raised by Seacole's officer friends/customers saw to it that she was able to live well and continued to be appreciated, if not celebrated, after her early years of fame.

Perhaps the most insidious in its effect is the use of Seacole myths in reading and grammar tests. The pupil must choose between alternative false statements to demonstrate comprehension or correct grammatical usage. For example, Macmillan Education English tests for Units 12 and 13 recount the Seacole (mythical) story, then ask pupils to circle True, False or Not Mentioned.[20] Another, for Level 4, tests pupils on the use of 'who' or 'which' using statements about Seacole that are erroneous.[21]

Since Seacole is taught in English schools, museums put on exhibitions and displays about her for school trips. They provide websites with 'resources' for teachers, which largely repeat the usual misinformation. For example, the Museum of London claims medical expertise for Seacole and her mother, including the use of 'English medicines to cure disease.' It employs medical symbols and references the Red Cross in connection with Seacole, who was neither a doctor nor had anything to do with the Red Cross. In fact, Red Cross founder, Henri Dunant, said that Nightingale was his inspiration.[22]

The campaign for a Mary Seacole statue was launched in 2003. In 2007, the Guy's and St Thomas' NHS Foundation Trust, without consultation, agreed to the statue's placement at its site. The statue committee is chaired by Lord Soley, a retired peer of Jamaican origin, with vice-chair Elizabeth Anionwu, CBE, a retired nursing professor,

---

[20] Macmillan English 6: Progress Test 6, Units 12 and 13, accessed 24 January 2014.

[21] Denis Vincent and Michael De la Mare, Michael, Effective Reading Tests: Mary Seacole Level 4. Macmillan Education 1986.

[22] Ellen Hart, *Man Born to Live: Life and Work of Henry Dunant, Founder of the Red Cross* 258.

Fellow of the Royal College of Nursing and a major source of points disputed here. In 2012, the Lambeth Planning Committee approved the installation of the statue at St Thomas'. The statue is to be larger than Nightingale's (at another location) and is to designate Seacole as a 'Pioneer Nurse.' The 'Nightingale Society' was formed in 2012 to counter the statue campaign and generally to answer the misinformation in circulation.

Geographically, while there is a substantial Jamaican component, the Seacole campaign's leaders, publications and websites have been overwhelmingly British. In a troubling trend, Americans have begun to join in uncritically and enthusiastically, contributing articles in *The New Yorker* and the *American Journal of Nursing* as well as a novel on Seacole.

At least ten doctoral dissertations have been produced at American universities in recent years, all of them repeating the core myths of heroism and pioneer nursing: one each in 2002, 2003, 2004, 2006 and 2011,[23] two in 1996,[24] and three in 2010.[25] Two British theses appeared in this period,

---

[23] Tate J. Hurvitz, Factually Speaking: The Rhetoric of Science and the Formation of Subjects in Victorian Writing, University of California, Riverside; Angelia Poon, Bodying Englishness Forth: Performing the English Subject and Colonialism in the Victorian Period, Brandeis; Jessica May Howell, Under the Weather: Disease, Race and Climate in Victorian Tales of Travel, University of California, Davis; Jessica Damian Schelke, The Lucid Silver and the Glowing Ore: British Women Writers Mine South America, 1770-1860, University of Miami; Alison Elizabeth McMonagle, The Wondrous Body of Mary Seacole: Mobility, Subjectivity and Display in a Transatlantic Life, George Washington University.

[24] Cheryl J. Fish, 'Going Mobile: The Body at Work,' Black and White Women's Travel Narratives, 1841-1857, City University of New York and Jessica Damian Schelke, The Lucid Silver and the Glowing Ore: British Women Writers Mine South America, 1770-1860, University of Miami.

[25] Brandy B. Fraley, From Dissection to Connection: The Preservative Power of the Empathetic Gaze in Romantic Literature, Ohio University; Bonnie McKay Harmer, Silenced in History: A Historical Study of Mary Seacole, University of Nebraska; Teddie Michelle Potter, Reconstructing a New Story of Nursing: Critical Analysis of Nursing Textbooks using Riane Eisler's Partnership Paradigm, California Institute of Integral Studies.

one highly critical of Nightingale that propagates the usual myths about Seacole. The other is considerably more sophisticated than any of the other theses, but still uncritically accepts the same key myths.[26] Doctoral theses of course lead to academic careers and further publications. Journal articles and chapters from several of these theses duly appear in Chapter 5, where the myths are refuted with primary source evidence — material conspicuously absent in the theses themselves.

The dissertation writers to date seem to have been stronger at emoting than finding reliable sources. One, for example, expressed 'disgust and shame' at the minimal inclusion of Seacole at the Florence Nightingale Museum,[27] although another complaint might be its trivializing of Nightingale and omission of her most significant work. Of course theses have advisors, committee members and examiners, so that one wonders about the general level of misinformation in academe generally. Many of the publications refuted in Chapter 5 are the work of reputable academics.

Seacole has also made it into the American nursing curriculum. For example, a graduate nursing course at Walden University, Minneapolis, presents Seacole as a pioneer of public health care and community health, and an innovative practitioner, linking her to Lillian Wald, an early American public health advocate. According to the course notes, Seacole had 'advanced practice nursing skills and administrative expertise' that 'set her apart' at a crucial time in history. There is no mention of Nightingale or her work on nursing or public health.[28]

---

[26] Christopher Middleton, Caring, Control and Compliance: Nursing's Struggle to be Audible, Univeristy of Nottingham, 2013; Anita Jacqueline Rupprecht, Civilised Sentience and the Colonial Subject: The Interesting Narrative of Olaudah Equiano or Gustavus Vassa, the African, and Wonderful Adventures of Mrs Seacole in Many Lands, University of Sussex, 2000.

[27] McMonagle, The Wondrous Body of Mary Seacole 3.

[28] Janol Montroy, Week 2: Reflection: Nursing Foundations of Community Health. Promoting and Preserving Health in a Diverse Society, Walden University NURS 6150, 2011.

How the tide has turned. Macmillan's 1913 official biography of Nightingale[29] is still the most comprehensive and accurate account of her life. That work is long out of print and Macmillan now publishes some of the most erroneous books on Seacole in its Education series. Cambridge University Press in the past was renowned for its tough peer-review process. Now it publishes works, which reveal uncritical acceptance of core Seacole myths. How did all those Doctors of Philosophy get it wrong?

A note on editing

Names of persons are spelled as per current usage or the correct name is inserted if an incorrect one appeared in a text. Abbreviations are normally written out in full. Dates are standardized to day, month, year. Punctuation and capitalization are modernized. First names and positions are added in square brackets where necessary. The spelling of place names is standardized, for example, Balaclava and Koulali.

Longer excerpts are set off from the main text and end with // All book sources are fully given in the References, authors' names and short titles in the text or footnotes. Ellipses by this author are indicated by ... while those in a quoted source are indicated by x x. Sources abbreviated as 'Add Mss' are British Library manuscripts.

Quotations not otherwise identified are from Seacole's memoir, the 1988 Oxford edition, abbreviated *WA* where necessary for clarity. References abbreviated *CW* are to Nightingale's work in Lynn McDonald, ed., *Florence Nightingale: The Crimean War*.

---

[29] Edward T. Cook, *The Life of Florence Nightingale*.

Timeline

The following timeline illustrates Mary Seacole's and Florence Nightingale's occupations and contributions to nursing and health care:[30]

Mary Seacole	Florence Nightingale
1805 Born in Kingston, Jamaica	
1820	Born in Florence, Italy
In the 1820s, two visits to England; on second visit, sells Jamaican pickles and preserves	
1836 Marries Edwin Seacole; together operate store in Black River; 'nurses' him and patroness in dying days	Experiences call to service, but family forbids her from pursuing nursing
1843 Mother's boarding house destroyed by fire, then rebuilt	1840s, visits workhouse infirmaries, which 'broke the visitor's heart'
1850 Travels to Panama, supervises food/clothing production for sale at brother's hotel/store; opens store/restaurant; cholera epidemic breaks out but no doctor is available; treats patients and claims some cures (uses lead acetate)	Makes first visit to Kaiserswerth Deaconess Institution, Germany
1851	Nurses three months at Kaiserswerth
1852	Seeks hospital experience in Dublin, but hospital closed for renovations

---

[30] Adapted from the timeline in Lynn McDonald, 'Florence Nightingale and Mary Seacole on Nursing and Health Care,' *Journal of Advanced Nursing* 69, 11 (November 2013). The items for Nightingale are necessarily selective, given the vast number known.

1853 Helps in yellow fever epidemic in Jamaica; no cure available; cares for dying grandmother at her home

Nurses for three months in Paris hospitals

From 1853 to 1854, nurses at and directs the Establishment for Gentlewomen during Illness (Harley St.)

1854 Returns to Panama; invests in gold mine, begins prospecting; leaves for London in September to attend to gold stocks

On October 21, leaves for Crimean War with 38 nurses

On November 5, arrives at Scutari; nurses at the Barrack Hospital; becomes superintendent of nursing at various hospitals

Late 1854, starts applying in person to be an 'army assistant' but does not submit application to be a nurse; reports rejection; forms plan with business partner to open 'mess table and comfortable quarters' for convalescent officers

Establishes laundries and kitchens; reports terrible conditions to war secretary, Sidney Herbert

1855 June 18, sells mule-loads of food and drink to spectators at Cathcart's Hill, watching 1st Redan assault; assists with first aid post-battle

In January/February, serious overcrowding at Scutari Barrack Hospital and rising death rates; new hospitals opened

On August 16, sells food and drink at the Battle of the Tchernaya; assists with first aid post-battle; cuts souvenir buttons off coats of dead Russian soldiers

In March, Sanitary Commisions arrives; Nightingale begins collaboration with Dr Sutherland

In May, makes first trip to Crimean hospitals; falls ill of 'Crimean fever' but recovers; convalesces; returns to Scutari

September 8, sells food and drink to spectators at 2nd Redan assault; assists with first aid post-battle

On October 8, makes a second visit to Crimea to establish nursing in its hospitals

September 9, borrows mules for catering; visits deserted Sebastopol; accepts loot from French soldiers stolen from Russian churches

On November 21, returns to Scutari on cholera epidemic outbreak;

From September 1855 to April 1856, caters excursions and sporting events; expands business during peace negotiations

During winter, continues nursing and supervision; writes letters to families on behalf of soldiers, providing information on their last care; continues to report to Sidney Herbert on need for reforms

1856 March 30, peace treaty signed; troops begin departure for England; stock cannot be sold; business fails

From March to May, makes third visit to Crimea; starts nursing at Land Transport Corps Hospital

In June, attends investiture for the Order of the Bath; sends a cake to officers

In April, officially named superintendent of all Crimean hospital nursing

In July, returns to England and is feted at dinners and public events; briefly runs store at Aldershot

Leaves Scutari on departure of last soldiers on July 28; arrives back in London on August 7

November 8, attends first bankruptcy court hearing, where Seacole first wears medals; fundraising begins

During September and October, visits queen at Balmoral Castle; meets Lord Panmure, secretary for war; agrees to write confidential account of war; starts statistical research

1857 January 17, bankruptcy certificate granted

Works on own reports and evidence for Royal Commission on the war

In July, publishes *Wonderful Adventures of Mrs Seacole in Many Lands*

Advises on nursing in the Royal Navy

Begins organizing first nurse training school

July 27, Surrey Gardens festival in Seacole's honour begins but proceeds meagre

1858 Visits Antwerp in July

Publishes *Notes on Matters affecting the Health of the British Army, Subsidiary Notes [on] the Introduction of Female Nursing into Military Hospitals*; writes papers for 1st edition of *Notes on Hospitals*;

1859 Henry Weekes produces sculpture of Seacole with medals (now at Getty Centre, Los Angeles); travels to Jamaica on the *Shannon*, arriving on October 13

Publishes *A Contribution to the Sanitary History of the British Army*; publishes expanded *Notes on Hospitals*

1860

In January, publishes *Notes on Nursing: What It Is, and What It Is Not*, which articulates principles of health promotion

	In June, Nightingale School of Nursing opens at St Thomas' Hospital, London
1861	Nightingale Ward and midwifery training open at King's College Hospital, London; Nightingale starts work on trained army nursing at Royal Victoria Hospital, Netley; publishes *Notes on Nursing for the Labouring Classes*; advises US government on Civil War hospitals; starts research on health conditions in India; census entry: 'formerly hospital matron'
1862	Advises on nursing in Baden, Germany; writes up research for Indian Royal Commission; advises on British army hospitals
1863 Visits Panama	Gives evidence to Royal Commission on India; publishes 'How People May Live and Not Die in India'
1864	Starts work on workhouse infirmary reforms; articulates principle of quality care for all, including those unable to pay; advises British delegation to Geneva Convention
1865 Returns to England in October on the *Atrato* from Jamaica	Trained nursing at Liverpool Workhouse begins; publishes Introduction to the *Organization of District Nursing*; writes 'Suggestions for a System of Nursing for Hospitals in India'
1866 In August, donates 100 bottles of anti-cholera medicine and 100 boxes of pills to Lord Mayor's Cholera Fund	Starts work on a system of nursing for Australia; works on extending workhouse nursing in London; advises on trained nursing for India
1867 In January, fundraising begins, which will support Seacole for rest of her life	Writes brief for Parliamentary Committee: 'Suggestions on...Training and Organizing Nurses for the Sick Poor in Workhouse Infirmaries'

1868		Nightingale nurses begin work in Sydney, Australia; Nightingale publishes 'Una and the Lion' on workhouse nursing; begins work to establish nursing at St Pancras Workhouse Infirmary
1869	Challen paints portrait of Seacole with three medals (now at National Portrait Gallery)	Works on nurses' housing at Netley and on Liverpool Workhouse nursing; analyses maternal mortality data at King's College Hospital
1870		Sends public letters to workhouse nurses; works on relief for Franco-Prussian War; publishes letter on cholera in *Lancet*
1871	Census entry from April: Seacole living in Paddington, London; occupation listed as 'annuitant'

In July, Gleichen terracotta bust completed of Seacole with four medals (now at Institute of Jamaica) | Census entry: occupation listed as 'director of Nightingale nurses'; Nightingale School moves to new St Thomas' Hospital; training school at St Pancras Workhouse Infirmary opens; Nightingale awarded Bronze Cross of French Aid Society; publishes *Introductory Notes on Lying-in Institutions* |
1872		Writes first address to nurses and students; advises on lectures for nurses at St Thomas'; trained nursing begins at Edinburgh Royal Infirmary
1873	Seacole carte de visite printed, with photograph wearing three medals, Maull & Co.	Works on St Thomas' curriculum and library for nurses; publishes 'Life or Death in India'; three American nurse training schools open based on Nightingale principles
1874		Begins work to send nurses to Montreal; advises on creation of a district nursing agency
1875		Works on army nursing; meets with nurses for Montreal; works on district nursing in Liverpool

1876	Begins mentoring matron at St Mary's, Paddington; Nightingale Fund begins support for district nurse training
1877	Extends district nursing; mentors matron at Addenbrooke's Hospital, Cambridge; publishes 'The Indian Famine'
1878	Works on nurses for Lincoln Infirmary, St Bart's, London, Herbert Hospital, Belfast and Kent; publishes 'The People of India'
1879	Starts inquiry on abuses in nursing at Buxton Hospital; advises on nursing in Austria; works on sending nurses to Anglo-Zulu War; publishes 'Woman Slavery in Natal'
1800	Mentors Manchester matron; advises on army nursing in southern Africa, workhouse infirmary nursing and district nursing
1881 Census entry from April: Seacole living in St Marylebone; occupation listed as 'independent' Dies on May 14	Census entry: occupation listed as 'director of Nightingale Fund for training hospital nurses;' advises on Metropolitan and National Nursing Association
1882	Works on nursing in India and Westminster Hospital, London; organizes nurses for Egyptian campaign
1883	Works on cholera in Egypt; nursing at Netley; plans for Nurses' Home at St Marylebone Workhouse
1884	Works on nurse training for Berlin; assists matron under investigation at St Mary's; Nurses' Home at St Marylebone Workhouse opens
1885	Works on nursing for new Egyptian campaign and for Belfast Children's

Hospital and Union Infirmary

1886	Works on nursing for Northern Hospital, Liverpool, India, Herbert Hospital, Jubilee Fund for District Nursing; publishes two articles in Quain, *Dictionary of Medicine*
1887	Selects and mentors new matrons at St Thomas' and Edinburgh Royal Infirmary; promotes nursing and health in home in India
1888	Advises on clinical lectures for probationers; works on district nursing for Scotland, midwifery nurse training, army nursing in India and nurses for Gordon Boys' Home; opposes proposal for state registration of nurses
1889	Mentors matrons of London Hospital and Birmingham Workhouse Infirmary; advises on nursing for London fever hospitals; assists matron and nurses going to Argentina
1890	New matron at St Thomas' appointed; publishes Introduction to Rathbone, *Sketch of the History and Progress of District Nursing*; advises on nursing in Baden and New Zealand
1891	Meets with Indian delegates at hygiene congress; publishes 'Sanitation in India;' census entry: occupation listed as 'director of Nightingale Fund Training School for Nurses'
1892	Works on district nursing in England and Scotland; mentors matron for Consumption Hospital; works on midwifery nursing; publishes on hospitals in *Chambers's Encyclopaedia* and 'The Reform of Sick Nursing and the Late Mrs Wardroper'

1893	Meets with American nursing leaders; assists on matron investigation at Radcliffe Infirmary
1894	Begins work on nurse training for Italy; publishes revised articles in Quain, *Dictionary of Medicine*
1895	Writes fundraising letter for St Thomas' Hospital; works with new medical instructor at Training School; organizes trained nurses for Bolton Workhouse Infirmary; begins work to establish trained nursing in Boston
1896	Works on nurse training for Finland; circulates Finnish procedures for aseptic surgery; advises on telephones and bells at St Thomas'; works on nursing for Irish workhouses and Calcutta; mentors matron of City of Dublin Hospital; publishes letter on district nursing
1897	Assists matron at London Hospital; assists matron at Edinburgh on investigation; advises nurses going to Hong Kong and India
1898	Tries to establish district nursing in Canada; does last work on health visitors; holds last meetings with St Thomas' nurses; makes last notes on antiseptic procedures
1899	Meets with matron of a New York hospital; meets with nursing leaders from Canada, US and New Zealand
1900	Last meetings with matrons of St Marylebone Workhouse and London Hospital; advises on nursing for Boer War; sends last 'address' (of 14) to nurses
1901	Sends public letter on district nursing; census entry: 'living on own means'

1902	Holds last meeting with matron of St Thomas' Hospital
1903	Sends letter on district nursing to Australia
1904	Has last meeting with a Kaiserswerth deaconess; sends last greetings to Australian nurses
1905	Sends last letter to Edinburgh Royal Infirmary nurses
1906	Meets with a midwife from Canada
1907	King confers Order of Merit on Nightingale; International Red Cross meeting recognizes her influence
1908	Sends last greetings to nurses and last message to survivors of the Light Brigade charge; City of London confers Freedom of City on her
1909	Holds last meeting with A.L. Pringle
1910	New building of Hospital for Gentlewomen opens; first Italian training school based on Nightingale principles opens in Rome
	Dies at home in London on August 13

Chapter 2

An overview of the Crimean War

The Crimean War (1854–56) was fought by the allies of Turkey, France and Britain against tsarist Russia, which was then menacing Europe by expanding its territory south of the Danube. The ostensible causes of the war were disputes over the control of sites in the Holy Land. France, under Emperor Napoleon III, was the chief instigator and sent by far the most troops. The emperor had immediate political objectives: to improve his support among Roman Catholics, who wanted more control of the holy sites, and — an old agenda item — to redress Napoleon I's terrible retreat on invading Russia half a century earlier. Lord Raglan, the British commander of the forces, had trouble remembering that the French were now his allies; he had been with Wellington at the Battle of Waterloo in 1815 when Napoleon I was finally, definitively defeated.[1]

The war did not start in the Crimea. When British and French troops began to leave for 'the East' in April 1854, they went first to Scutari (now Uskudar) on the Asiatic side of Constantinople (now Istanbul) and were next sent to Varna, in what is now Bulgaria. Russian encroachment into Bulgaria, 'south of the Danube,' had prompted the European nations to join Turkey, which had its own motives after the Russians sank its fleet in 1853. Then, early in 1854, the Russians drew their forces back north of the Danube, removing the most salient cause

---

[1] Colin Robins, annot., *The Murder of a Regiment: Winter Sketches from the Crimea* 31.

of the war. The British and French, however, instead of going home, made the conquest of Sebastopol, the major Russian harbour on the Black Sea, their goal. They expected to be in and out quickly. They made no preparations for a winter campaign.

Both the British and French had other reasons for needing to get out of Bulgaria in the summer of 1854, for both armies lost large numbers of men to cholera before a shot was fired. They sailed to the Crimean peninsula in early September 1854 and landed without opposition. Over the next three months, they fought three major battles: the Alma, Balaclava and Inkermann, moving progressively closer to Sebastopol. After Inkermann, on 5 November 1854, they settled in for what would become a ten-month siege, camped before Sebastopol.

Today's commentators on the Crimean War often assume that the conditions were more like World War I: a network of trenches with the two sides dug in for months or years, facing each other across a no-man's land, where the brave ventured out to rescue the wounded and remove the dead. In the Crimean War, the allies used trenches, while the Russians stayed within their fortified city, rebuilding the earthen fortifications by night that the allies bombarded by day. The siege of Sebastopol was never complete, so that the Russians could bring in supplies and leave as they wished. The trenches were miserable places; many men suffered from frostbite or were injured or killed by Russian shooting. Conditions for the men continued to be harsh even when on leave from the trenches, for there was no shelter apart from tents the first winter.

Shots were exchanged on occasion. Anyone walking in or near the camps was somewhat vulnerable, but people got used to occasional shells going by. The allies bombarded Sebastopol heavily for days before assaults and caused a lot of damage. By the end of the siege, the city had been largely destroyed, although the allies did not know how much damage they had done until they walked in.

All the battles were short, over within the day. In the case of the first failed attempt to take the Redan bastion of the Sebastopol fortification, one officer said that the attack began at 3:45 a.m. on 18 June 1855, while the 'sad finale' was at 7 a.m. He noted it was their 'first reverse.'[2]

There is a massive and growing amount of secondary literature on the Crimean War. Many officers kept journals and their families held on to their letters. Memoirs and correspondence began to come out as early as 1855 and continue to be published by descendants. Nightingale and her nurses get occasional mentions, Seacole fewer, typically by way of a passing note.

Nightingale's work on the Crimean War is the subject of a 1074-page volume in the *Collected Works of Florence Nightingale (CW)*. It is also the subject of a chapter in the short *Florence Nightingale at First Hand*, which gives highlights from the *Collected Works*. A well-edited volume of 100 letters by Nightingale was produced by Sue Goldie, *'I have Done my Duty': Florence Nightingale in the Crimean War*.

The material to be extracted here, however, draws on sources not already conveniently available: newspaper articles, letters and memoirs from the time, all by authors other than Nightingale or Seacole. This enables the reader to get a picture of the war and the roles that Nightingale and Seacole played in it by those who saw them in action. We begin with an account by Charles H. Bracebridge, a Nightingale family friend who, with his wife, accompanied Nightingale and her nurses to the East. On his return to England, he spoke publicly about the bad conditions he had seen, remarks that were widely circulated in the press. Nightingale was unhappy about the publicity, which made her life more difficult, but Bracebridge's account serves to show the reality they faced on arrival at Scutari. The extract also introduces the chef Alexis Soyer who worked with Nightingale on improving food for the soldiers.

From: 'Mr Bracebridge on the Crimean Hospitals,' *The Times* 16 October 1855 5F

When they [Nightingale and the nurses] first made their appearance at Scutari, there was neither kitchen, coals, nor candles — nothing in fact but the naked walls. They soon set to work, however, to make the place

---

[2] George Paget, *The Light Cavalry Brigade of the Crimea* 101–02.

comfortable, and in two days they effected a great change in the interior appearance of the building. They had at one time nearly 3,000 sick and wounded, and, if the beds had been placed at full length, they would have extended three miles and 500 yards. Many of the assistant surgeons — very young men — were attacked with fever from sleeping in the corridors that ran round the hospital. These rooms were so situated that, when fires were lighted in them, the draught brought all the impure air of the hospital into them, causing fever and other diseases....

When the band of female nurses first arrived, they were despised for their want of medical skill and disliked for their womanly curiosity, but two or three days after, when 600 wounded men were brought down, they dressed the wounds of 300 of them and waited upon them with the utmost tenderness and assiduity. The medical men then began to think they might be of some use....

But when M Soyer came out things went on much better. The meat, before he made his arrangements, was so bad that the men ate part of it raw and buried the remainder in the trenches. The men had no fuel or proper means of cooking, and, from their excessive work in the trenches, were not able to go in search of fuel to cook their meal. The French were much more expert at making a fire and cooking victuals, and they always managed so well that every man had a cup of hot coffee from a boiling cauldron before he went to the trenches, and a meal of bread and soup on his return.//

Senior chaplain, J.E. Sabin, provided his account of the dire conditions to the Cumming-Maxwell Commission, which conducted the first of the several investigations on the army hospitals.

From: J.E. Sabin, UK, *Report upon the State of the Hospitals of the British Army in the Crimea and Scutari* 314

I have been here [Scutari] since last July. I was present when the first wounded arrived. I think it was on Sunday, but we had a large batch of sick on Friday. There was a great want in the Barrack Hospital of bedsteads and beds. The sick and wounded were put into the wards;

some, not all, had beds, many without them. When the wounded arrived, they all had to lie on the floor. Corridors B and C were filled with men lying down; some had straw beds, but the majority were without anything under them, some without even a coat....The surgeons attended to them as fast as they could, but it was impossible to attend to them all....I was in every corner of the hospital every day. Whenever I was called to a dying man, I went.//

The autobiography of Cyrus Hamlin, a Protestant missionary to Turkey who was on the scene before the nurses arrived, includes both descriptions of the horrors of the hospital when it opened, and the challenges it faced providing basic food like bread. A bakery was established in Constantinople to provide jobs for poor Christian Armenians. It produced a good yeast bread, not the Turkish flat bread. Lord Raglan, the commander of the British forces, personally approved it and the bakery got the contract to supply the Barrack Hospital, only to lose it when Hamlin refused to pay a share of the profits to Dr Menzies, the principal medical officer, and the purveyor, as was customary (330). Dr Menzies was in effect Nightingale's boss and made life difficult for her, as Hamlin attests in his autobiography.

Losing the contract turned out to be lucky for the mission bakery, for the price of flour shot up by 50 % and the accommodating bakery that next got the contract suffered serious losses (332). The French brought their own bakers with them and produced good bread throughout the war. Hamlin also recorded Menzies's recall to England, on being discovered to have 'plundered the government enormously' (335).

From: Cyrus Hamlin, *My Life and Times* 329 and 332–34

The rapid filling up of the hospital by invalids and the wounded sent down from the front occasioned enormous evils that prudence and foresight should have prevented. Vessels were arriving almost every day, with fifty or a hundred or two hundred cases, and this rapid increase was not met by any corresponding increase of surgeons and nurses. The chief physician, Dr Menzies...was a selfish, greedy, beastly fellow, who seemed to think that, if the English soldier is given beer and brandy enough, he will do. The death rate was awful. The trenches were dug in the daytime, the burials were at night to avoid a panic.

Men were dying; some were dead and the sheet drawn over the face. The smells and sights were awful and I turned back, but seeing in one of the rooms a fine-looking soldier, raised to a half-sitting posture, I saluted him and asked him what they needed most. 'O Sir,' he said, 'night watchers. The lights are put out at nine or ten, and we are told "Every man is to be quiet and go to sleep." But after a time there is a cry for "Water, water!" and one is crazy and sings, another curses; some get up to help a comrade and are made worse by it, and so the long night wears away.' I offered to organize a night-watching corps of volunteers, but Dr Menzies rejected the offer with disdain.

It was just at this time that Florence Nightingale came, with a dozen trained nurses and forty hospital servants....I went one morning to the hospital to settle some accounts. When the business was finished, the purveyor said to me: 'Fancy, Mr Hamlin, some *women* have come to the hospital! A Miss Nightingale, with a force of assistants, has come and taken possession of rooms at the right of the front entrance. Was anything ever more improper than women in such a place?'

I replied: 'It is time, Mr Parker, that somebody should come in here and *do something*, for I do not believe that any Turkish hospital since the Turks took Constantinople ever equalled this in disorder, filth and suffering.'

'I know it, I know it,' he said, 'but we are soon to have surgeons and servants from England, and the things you have seen will soon be remedied. But these women will not stay long.' Dr Menzies set himself to make her position insufferable.//

The bakery contract had already been cancelled when Nightingale and her nurses arrived at Scutari and the new contractor produced bad bread. Complaints about it appear in the next excerpt, by the superior of the Bermondsey Sisters of Mercy, and even stronger complaints can be found in the journals of the Irish Sisters of Mercy. The story is picked up again when Nightingale, on visiting the small hospital at Koulali, found out that it had excellent bread — the contract with the mission bakery was still in force there — and demanded that the good bread be supplied also to the Barrack Hospital.

As the superior of the Bermondsey sisters described it:

Their food was so bad and so sparing that they were often faint from hunger--the bread was sour and often mouldy—the meat was of the worst description...the want of water was a suffering greater than can be expressed....Even for washing so little water was to be had, and so destitute were they of all conveniences, that they were forced to wash in the same water and in the same basin to wash also their linen.[3]

The next item, from the same frank account, shows unequivocally the failure of the hospital authorities to prepare for the nurses' arrival.

From: Notes of Mary Clare Moore, Bermondsey Annals, courtesy of Dr. Mary C. Sullivan, RSM

[November 1854]
It is scarcely possible to describe the extreme desolateness of these apartments. The room given to our sisters had no furniture except an old chair without a back, which served them for a table. The windows, completely broken, admitted the piercing air, for it was then bitterly cold and there was no means of procuring a fire. The commandant, Major Sillery, most kindly sent in mattresses and such bed covering as could be spared, and the soldiers gave part of their rations, no provisions having been laid in for this unforeseen addition....

A can of warm water therefore from the barrack kitchen was procured into which some tea was put and a small cup full, without milk or sugar, was measured into copper basins for each; this with a scanty portion of bread was their supper and this kind of privation, which they felt the more on account of their feverish state after such a trying journey, continued for many months. x x

---

[3] Mary C. Sullivan, ed. *The Friendship of Florence Nightingale and Mary Clare Moore* 54.

The purveyors were unwilling to place the hospital stores and clothing at Miss Nightingale's disposal. However, before the end of the first week, she succeeded in obtaining leave to send nurses to the General Hospital, a building similar in design to the Barrack, the number of patients being above a thousand. The distance was about a mile over a bleak rocky hill, beset with wild dogs....

Rev Mother with Sister M. Stanislaus and Sister M. de Chantal had work in some of the wards of the Barrack Hospital when suddenly the news of the fatal engagement at Inkermann came, and this was quickly followed by crowds of wounded men in the worst stage of destitution on the 9th November and the succeeding days. The sisters were now almost overworked preparing the wards and beds and, according as the wounded arrived, helping them, dressing their wounds and comforting them. The want of changes of linen being one of the greatest miseries, Miss Nightingale undertook to have the soldiers' shirts washed and mended and she purchased a supply of shirts and flannels, the men having all lost their kits on the field. They had also been without the means of washing themselves for weeks and were, therefore, in a most sad state, so that those employed for them in any way were covered with vermin.//

The 'extremely sour' bread was also a complaint of an Anglican sister, who included this detail in a letter that also blasted the care given by doctors at the hospital. She was forced to leave after the letter appeared in *The Times*.[4]

A captain of the Artillery visiting the Barrack Hospital in January 1855, the month with the highest death rate, recorded the horrors of what he saw.

---

[4] Letter of Elizabeth Wheeler 11 November 1854, published in *The Times* 8 December 1854 8D.

From: E. Bruce Hamley, *The Story of the Campaign of Sebastopol, Written in the Camp* 150–51

[January 1855]

Entering any of the corridors or wards, the same scene presented itself. The occupants of some of the beds sat strongly up, eating heartily their soup and meat; others, emaciated to skeletons, more like corpses than living beings, except for the large, hollow, anxious eyes, lay back on their pillows, or tried with difficulty to swallow the spoonfuls of arrowroot or sago offered to them by the attendants. There seemed no doubtful class — all were broadly marked either for life or death....At some beds a woman, the wife of the patient, sat chatting with him; beside others stood the somewhat ghostly appearance of a Catholic Sister of Charity, upright, rigid, veiled and draped in black; the veil projecting far beyond her face threw it, as well as the white linen folded cross her bosom, into deep shadow. The thinness of some of the forms propped up against their pillows, their chests exposed by the open shirts, was absolutely frightful; the bony hands wandered vaguely about the hair and sunken temples, and the eyes were fixed on vacancy. Some lay already in the shadow of death, their eyes reverted, showing only the whites beneath the drooping lids, and others had passed this last stage, and waited only for the grave.//

The same Artillery captain noted the improvements in food made by the nurses:

> In the great kitchen, close by their quarter, rice pudding, manufactured on a grand scale, was transferred, smoking, by an enormous ladle to the destined platters; beef-tea and mutton broth were being cooked in huge caldrons ... and flocks of poultry were simmering into boiled fowls or chicken broth (152).

These reforms, however, were superficial and could do nothing to alleviate the suffering of the resigned 'skeletons.' The Sanitary Commission did not arrive until March, 1855.

The next two extracts are from J.C. MacDonald who was in charge of the *Times* Fund which Nightingale used for purchasing needed supplies.

From: Our own correspondent, 'The Sick and Wounded Fund,' *The Times* 29 January 1855 10A

Winter has at length descended upon the Bosphorus, bearing on its pinions a more than usual load of cheerlessness and gloom.... These vast establishments, which require so much the general superintendence of one sensible, vigorous head, still remain in this respect as they were nearly three months ago, when their defective state and the consequent sufferings of their inmates first awakened attention at home.

What has been done during that considerable interval can be very easily stated. Miss Nightingale and her nurses and sisters have, with the aid of the Fund which I administer, filled up the worst and largest gaps in their administration. By them the shortcomings in the purveyors' department have been compensated, the defects of the orderly system in some degree palliated, and urgent wants provided for, which otherwise must have been left entirely unsupplied....

I have said that what has been done in the hospitals has been done mainly by temporary expedients, but I have not stated that, in spite of these, they are daily becoming more crowded, more in a state dangerous to life, more entirely every day huge, disorderly, ill-arranged lazar [fever] houses, without any classification of patients or any systematic distribution of hospital *matériel*....

Far from aspiring to having each bed supplied with its own set of utensils, body clothing, bedding, etc., as in the French service, our humble-minded military surgeon trembles to ask for the requisite boards and trestles to raise his patients off the floor. As for clean linen, though the patients be dysenteric, and brought on shore pasted over with their own excrement, that is a luxury which the purveyor-in-chief, when he has any in store, gives out as a miser parts with his gold....

All these evils exist, and will continue to do so, complicating each other, until a remedy sufficiently sweeping and comprehensive to embrace them all is supplied. The extraordinary powers given to the ambassador [Lord Stratford de Redcliffe] have failed to do so, and are a dead letter. The commission of inquiry [Cumming-Maxwell], which was made such a handle of in Parliament, has been equally fruitless, and has the doom of most other commissions clearly stamped on it. Lord William Paulet [commandant of the Bosphorus], after a few incipient manifestations of vigour, has relapsed into the mere depot commandant, and is obviously frightened at the task before him should he venture one inch further in setting matters straight than the rules of the service render necessary.//

From: Our own correspondent, *The Times* 1 February 1855 8D-E

Eleven hundred more sick are on their way here [Scutari] from the Crimea, and the latest news received thence affords no ground for hoping that the amount of disease and mortality in the army is on the decline. On the contrary, there is every reason to fear that both are increasing, for the weather is now dreadfully severe, with heavy snow one day and biting frost the next....We have already in hospital from thirty to forty cases of mortified feet from exposure, and the spectacle which men thus afflicted present is far more distressing than the severest wounds. It is remarkable how, on cold and stormy nights, the deaths here run up, and another singular feature is the extent to which on such nights the dysenteric patients rave....

We have now on the Bosphorus and Dardanelles no less than eight hospitals, containing an aggregate of nearly 5,000 sick and wounded. The largest, and by far the most important of these, is the Barrack Hospital, which holds from 2,000 to 3,000 patients (all of them severe cases) and which is partitioned off into three divisions, each under the care of a first-class staff surgeon. Next in size to the Barrack Hospital is the General Hospital, also filled with cases requiring active treatment and superintendence by two senior medical officers....

Koulali, on the Bosphorus, was originally appropriated to the Russian wounded, but they are to be removed to the arsenal at Stamboul, and our own sick have already taken their places to the number of 350 or 400.//

Many of the nuns in the new contingent were placed at Koulali, when the barrack there was turned into a hospital. It opened in January 1855, initially under the superintendence of Mary Stanley, who wrote a reminiscence of the experience on visiting the area seven years later. She did not mention, nor did other sources of the time, that the Koulali Hospital had the highest death rate of all the war hospitals, due to the unsanitary conditions. It, like the others, was cleaned up by the Sanitary Commission. When Stanley left, Mother Mary Francis Bridgeman of the Irish Sisters of Mercy succeeded her as superintendent.

From: Mary Stanley, 'Ten Days in the Crimea,' *Macmillan's Magazine* 5 February 1862: 302–03

In January [1855] we began work at the hospital at Koulali. There we realized what protracted war was. The battles were over. It was not the wounded we were called upon to tend, but those who were stricken down with fever, dysentery and frostbites, from long exposure in the trenches....

Some days and scenes are specially stamped upon one's memory. Who will forget the arrival of the first batch of invalids who were to be located in the upper hospital only vacated by the Turks a week before? The huge wood fire in the stoveless kitchen, the large caldrons of water set on, the basins of arrowroot mixed, thrown in and stirred with a long wooden pole, for want of better implements! Then was the melancholy procession up the hill: worn-out men dragging their weak and weary frames along, some supported on each side, some carried on stretchers....

Besides the mournful sight of the processions of the sick, there was daily the still sadder sight of the dead, borne away from the dead-house in the centre of the court to the cemetery on the hillside. At 3 or 4 o'clock each afternoon, the chaplain was in attendance there to read the service over the one large grave....

Where any relation was present, a coffin was granted. A sheet from the stores was thrown over it, and it was borne by four soldiers. And, deep in mud, we toiled up the hill. Most impressively the funeral service was read. It was a most affecting sight; the words of the service, the associations, the rudeness of the external of the mourners, the deep grief of the poor woman [the widow Stanley was accompanying], the group close by filling up the daily pit with its twelve uncoffined dead, the glorious view of Constantinople across the Bosphorus!//

The laundry

Cyrus Hamlin, the American missionary whose mission bakery produced good bread for the hospitals, did another great service in establishing the laundry at Koulali. He discovered that the men's clothing was so loaded with vermin that the soldiers preferred to suffer from the cold rather than wear it (356). Crimean lice were 'large, fat, disgusting, overgrown, *hellish-looking creatures,*' which punctured the skin, causing inflammation and intolerable burning: 'I have no doubt they killed more English soldiers than all the Russian bullets' (358). The clothes in the army stores were as bad as what the men had on.

He asked the chief physician why washing was not done, not even for patients who had been there for two weeks. The doctor explained that the Greek women employed to wash, who used the salt water of the Bosphorus, brought the clothes back damp, which killed the men 'quicker than anything else' (357). Hamlin pointed out that there were many unemployed people willing to work and was told to mind his business. In due course he got copper kettles set in masonry and pumps going.

From: Cyrus Hamlin, *My Life and Times* 360

The truth was, the clothes were so filthy, disgusting and loaded with vermin that the women feared to touch them, and declared they would never enter the place again. About three thousand articles had been brought over, in large bundles, and opened in the court, and the offensive odour had gone up into the windows of the houses on that side. The people, naturally excited, were assembling in angry haste. Here was trouble all around! I told the people their complaints were reasonable, and the clothes should be immediately removed to the magazine on the other side....What was I to do? I was certainly in a *fix*. I could not blame the women or the people.//

He assembled a team of workmen he knew, and plunged in himself. They now had adequate soap and hot water, and the new equipment worked. The soapy water ran off filthy and muddy, then the clothes were rinsed with pure water and came out transformed (361). The women employees returned. The doctor who had been a 'brutal, unfeeling wretch' was removed and replaced by Dr Tice, who had revealed the conspiracy about the bread contract to Hamlin. As soon as a complete set of clean clothing could be supplied, it was sent to the hospital, which produced 'joy and comfort' in the men. Dr Tice then ordered the patients to change clothes twice a week (362).

Regimental hospitals

A surgeon with the Light Infantry described the terrible state of a (typical) regimental hospital early in the war after visiting one with a colleague upon his arrival at the front on 5 February 1855. The regimental hospitals kept the less serious cases, transferring the more serious cases to the general hospitals at Scutari.

From: Douglas Arthur Reid, *Memories of the Crimean War* 9

Naturally, I expected to see a hut or building of some kind and was much astonished when he pointed out a row of bell tents pitched, like all the others, in the mud. I looked into some of them and found them crowded with sick, ten or twelve men in each tent with their feet towards the pole and their heads towards the curtain. They were lying on the bare ground wrapped in their great coats. It struck me that, whatever was the matter with them, they had a very poor chance of recovery. They were being sent down daily in batches to Balaclava for embarkation to Scutari or England. The diseases from which they suffered were chiefly dysentery and fever. The regiment had then been more than two months in camp, and this was the best they could do for their sick and wounded!//

As the next extract shows, the surgeon was not much pleased either when huts were erected to replace the tents. Reid did not publish his memoir until 1911, so he was able to add perspective after acquiring knowledge of antiseptics. Joseph Lister's great breakthrough, antiseptic surgery, took place a decade too late for the Crimean War (he began his experiments in 1865, publishing in 1867). Anaesthetics had only recently come into use but were resisted by some doctors, notably Dr John Hall.

From: Douglas Arthur Reid, *Memories of the Crimean War* 40–41

Lord Raglan paid a surprise visit to our camp hospital after the huts had been erected. He expressed himself as much pleased with its equipment and with the kind of huts supplied. I cannot say that we were satisfied. That they were an improvement upon the tents previously used as a hospital there can be no question, but the huts were constructed of thin boards, and the roofs were not protected by felt and, consequently, were not weatherproof. As to the equipment, the supply of medical and surgical necessaries was meagre in the extreme, and, as to medical comforts, there were none. We could not get proper diet for the patients, nor could anything be cooked properly.

An order came out that as many sick as possible should be sent away home and not detained at Scutari, where the hospitals were becoming overcrowded. This was a sensible arrangement, as it enabled us to keep our regimental hospital more free for the reception of recent casualties, which were coming in continually.

Some of the wounded men were dreadfully troubled by the flies that, in spite of all precautions, managed to get to their wounds, with the result that, very often, on removing the dressings, we found them full of maggots. It must be borne in mind that antiseptic treatment was not available fifty-five years ago, for the simple reason that our present-day antiseptics were unknown. We managed to kill the maggots by filling the wounds with calomel [mercury chloride], which happened to be one of the drugs of which we had a plentiful supply, and for which we had little other use. The water that we used to *cleanse* the wounds was by no means free from impurities, so that there was ample reason for getting the poor fellows out of camp as soon as they could be moved.//

MP Augustus Stafford, who made a private visit to Turkey early in the war, later gave evidence to the Roebuck Committee on the state of the Barrack Hospital. Bowel diseases were responsible for roughly half the hospital deaths at the time. Nightingale presumably never was in the men's toilets, so she quoted his description in her (here abbreviated) *Notes on the Health of the British Army* (full title: *Notes on Matters Affecting the Health, Efficiency and Hospital Administration of the British Army*, reprinted in *CW* 706–07). A 'necessary' is a toilet, or, in this case, a slab with an opening into a tile pipe leading to a sewer under the building.

From: Evidence of Augustus Stafford to the Roebuck Committee, *First Report from the Select Committee of the Army Before Sebastopol*. 1854–55 vol IX, para 7523

19 March 1855

When the barrack was re-opened as a hospital, no sufficient pains were taken to repair those pipes, or secure a flow of water, and the pipes soon choked up, and the liquid feces, the evacuations from those afflicted with diarrhea, filled up the pipes, floated up over the floor, and came into the room in which the necessaries were, extended and flowed into the anteroom, and were more than an inch deep when I got there in the morning; men suffering from diarrhea, who had no slippers at the time and no shoes on as this flood of filth advanced, came less and less near to the necessary, and nearer and nearer to the door, till at last I found them within a yard of the anteroom performing the necessary functions of nature, and, in consequence, the smell from this place was such that I can use no epithet to describe its horror....

The hideous state of the privies, too truly described in this last extract, which refers to the Barrack Hospital, continued there, more or less, up to March 1855, in which month it was still occasionally at once our crime and our punishment. A farther misery, and the cause of much disease, was, in the autumn of 1854, the placing of tubs in those wards farthest from the privies (in the absence of utensils [bedpans]), to hold the excreta of from thirty to fifty patients afflicted with diarrhea and dysentery; it is easy to imagine the consequence of this frightful nuisance, and it often became Miss Nightingale's duty to see these tubs removed and emptied by a couple of orderlies, who carried one on a pole between them. These tubs were, however, discontinued at a late period of the winter of 1854–55.//

Officers and ordinary soldiers

The gap in privileges (and responsibilities) between officers, on the one hand, and non-commissioned officers (sergeants and corporals) and ordinary soldiers (privates), on the other, remains great. It was vastly greater at the time of the Crimean War. Nightingale's concern was to improve conditions for ordinary soldiers, who were expected, by most of their officers, to live and act like brutes, and who, recruited from the poorest of the land, were accustomed to harsh conditions. Flogging was still used as a punishment. Ordinary rations for soldiers were salt beef or salt pork, with hard biscuit instead of bread. Rice and vegetables were introduced gradually by reformers. Lime juice was supplied to soldiers only when evidence of scurvy became all too obvious (the navy had been using this remedy for years). Soap was not issued to the men until nearly a year after the troops arrived, although bowel diseases were rampant, running water was not available and the toilet areas were overflowing. The men wanted soap and eagerly washed, Nightingale reported, when they got it.

The daily ration of a soldier at the end of April 1856, when improvements had been made, was: 1¼ lbs fresh or 1 lb salt meat; 1½ lb fresh bread or 1 lb biscuit; 1 oz coffee or ¼ oz tea, 2 oz sugar, 2 oz rice; 1 oz lime juice; and salt and pepper.[5]

The daily alcohol allowance provided by the army to soldiers was initially 1 gill, or 5 oz, later reduced to ½ gill, on the recommendation of the Sanitary Commission and a board of officers (231). The same alcohol ration was provided to the Turkish troops, most of whom sold theirs to British soldiers, resulting in 'no small injury of the latter.' Brandy was liberally furnished prior to battle, especially to the infantry, to make them reckless. Benefactors sent special gifts, such as local draft beer, to their regiments.

Soldiers could augment their food and drink by purchases at a canteen, which was run typically by a merchant or 'sutler,' often Italian, Greek or Levantine. Canteens were grouped together in 'bazaars.' As an extract has already mentioned, the French had better food (and coffee) provided by the army than the British. Their cantonières were also better, as an extract will shortly show.

The contrasting conditions experienced by men and officers in hospital can be nicely seen in the next extract, which is taken from notes made by an officer of the Royal Engineers when he was a patient at the Palace Hospital for diarrhea, or 'the prevalent Crimean disorder,' as he called it. The hospital consisted of two buildings, run entirely distinctly: the smaller quarters for officers and a larger building for the men. The setting was idyllic: 'one of the prettiest spots in the Bosphorus,' the sea 'deep pellucid blue,' the 'bright green foliage' and 'quaint Eastern architecture, picturesque costumes, tranquillity and beauty.' This was when ordinary soldiers at the Scutari Barrack Hospital were placed on thin straw mats on a stone floor, 18 inches apart, in overcrowded wards and corridors, badly lacking ventilation and sanitary facilities.

---

[5] John Sutherland, *Report of the Sanitary Commission* 230.

From: Whitworth Porter, *Life in the Trenches* 183–86

I was speedily ushered into a room of which, as the hospital was not much crowded, I was to be the sole occupant: a cool, cheerful room it was — a corner room with windows running along two sides of it, all opened wide ... a gentle breeze was playing, rendering it, to my wearied and feverish senses, a very paradise indeed. A divan stretched along the whole of one side of the room beneath the windows; beside it stood my bed, whose snow-white sheets and well-stuffed mattress seemed to speak most eloquently of rest. The room was provided with every requisite for an officer's bedroom, and on the table in the centre stood a little vase filled with fresh-culled flowers, evidently placed there to greet the weary wanderer on his first arrival....

The arrangements for the comfort of the sick officers in this hospital were in every way admirable....Each officer paid one shilling per day for his messing, and for this trifling sum he was provided with every comfort and even luxury necessary to his condition. His day's ration consisted of half a fowl, half a pound of mutton, five eggs and a due provision of tea, sugar, milk, bread, etc., in addition to which the doctor had unlimited powers to order wine, beer or spirits, in any quantity he might think proper....There were also stores untold of medical comforts such as sago, arrowroot, chocolate, jelly, sweet biscuits, etc., all of which might be obtained by the mere asking....

Such of the officers as were not too sick dined together at a mess; the entire of the crockery, plate, linen and glass were provided by Lady Stratford de Redcliffe [wife of the British ambassador to Turkey]....She also presented each officer with a small service for breakfast and tea, sufficient for two persons, which he kept in his own room.//

Further details this officer gave include the arrival of soap, eau de cologne and cold cream, sent by the queen. Life was comfortable, if monotonous. His servant brought him breakfast when he wanted it and the doctor visited at 10 o'clock. There was a reading room 'amply supplied with both papers and periodicals,' and a garden for lounging (186–88).

Spectators and helpers

The Crimean War, like others of its time but unlike wars of today, attracted spectators. 'Travelling gentlemen,' known as 'TGs,' officers' wives, war correspondents and foreigners watched from a convenient, high-up spot. Henri Dunant, founder of the Red Cross, had his first glimpse of war as a spectator at the Battle of Solférino in 1859, invited by Napoleon III, whom he had gone to see on a matter of business.

Providing refreshments to these spectators was a regular business. This was presumably Seacole's plan on her arrival at Balaclava, as suggested by a story in *The Times*: 'I suppose the lady calculates on a liberal share of the patronage when the excursion visitors come out to the siege in the summer.'[6]

Dr Reid, in his memoir quoted above, noted that sutlers, 'who sold goods (mostly food and drink), ... were present in great numbers in Balaclava and Kadikoi' (13–14). The French Army was better organized, with a 'cantonière' attached to each section, where extra food and drink could be bought.[7]

Officers' wives came out to the war for various lengths of time and they visited the local scenes. An extract from Soyer's *Culinary Campaign* describes a French sentry pointing out that ladies 'often came to this spot to get a view' and that he had 'never known the enemy to fire while they were present' (174).

Lady George Paget, the beautiful young wife of Lord George Paget, was a favourite of Lord Raglan's, accompanying him on horseback on his tours — she was the only woman at his bedside when he died. During her stay she became 'the toast of the army' and 'while the carnage continued, she and her fashionable friends picnicked, dined, danced, went on conducted tours of the battlefields, attended parades and reviews [and] patronised the race meetings.' The British ambassador to Turkey, Lord

---

[6] 'The Siege of Sebastopol,' *The Times* 9 March 1855 9E.

[7] Robins, annot., *The Murder of a Regiment* 18.

Stratford de Redcliffe, also 'brought a party of ladies and gentlemen from Constantinople to tour the front.'[8]

Spectators also helped when they could. Officers' wives, notably Lady George Paget, visited the sick and wounded men at the Balaclava hospital. Seacole noted that war correspondent W.H. Russell found time, 'even in his busiest moment, to lend a helping hand to the wounded' on the battlefield (*WA* 171). Shepherd commented that 'certain women even went up to the advanced lines, often under fire, to render first aid or to help bring in the wounded,' naming Seacole as being in 'a special category' (506). Indeed, 'many appeared on the field of battle to succour the wounded and one was found to be assisting a surgeon while he operated' (90–91).

People back home, as soon as they heard about the bad conditions, began to send parcels, all of which had to be acknowledged, whether they were of use or not. The *Times* Fund made available to Nightingale to purchase goods was enormously useful while the well-meant parcels could be a terrible nuisance.

Elizabeth Herbert, wife of the secretary at war and a friend of Nightingale's, wrote about the problem of sending parcels, an issue that early on indicated how bad the army's organization was.

From: Letter of Elizabeth Herbert to Parthenope Nightingale, Claydon House bundle 272

17 November [1854]

As to the parcels for Scutari, *it's no use sending them in the transports,* and I grieve to say we do not now see a hope of the *Ottawa* packages being delivered till they have been to Balaclava. The necessity for troops is so urgent that they must go direct to the Crimea and the captain, if he stopped at Constantinople, would not 'break bulk.' Sidney therefore is engaging a steamer through Dr Smith to go straight to Scutari with medical stores, and in that packet

---

[8] John Shepherd, *The Crimean Doctors: A History of the British Medical Services in the Crimean War* 506.

your boxes can go. Send them all to me, and send also a fresh supply of clothes, flannel, socks, knitted jackets, etc., for alas! the *Ottawa* stores may not reach them for months.//

Cholera and other bowel diseases

The three great bowel diseases that afflicted so many soldiers, doctors and others during the Crimean War were cholera (in two epidemics), diarrhea and dysentery (in larger numbers but lower death rates). None of these diseases had been conclusively identified at this point and there was no known cure for any of them. (Using current medical language, diarrhea is not a disease but a group of diseases caused by different bacteria or parasites — all characterized by fluid discharge of the bowel. Dysentery is more severe diarrhea, with blood or mucus, and is now identified as two types: amoebic, discovered in 1875, and the more severe bacillary, discovered in 1898.)

Cholera was the deadliest of the three, at the time killing roughly 50–60 % of those treated, often within a few hours of onset. The disease is now known to be caused by a bacillus that thrives in the bowel and is transmitted by fecal-laden water. German bacteriologist Robert Koch conclusively identified it only in 1883.

Cholera arrived in Britain in the early 1830s. Doctors experimented with treatments, using an array of toxic substances considered helpful for their effect of purging the system, notably mercury chloride and lead acetate. Medical journals and books of 'materia medica' advocated the use of these toxic chemicals, sometimes, though not often, with cautions. It was not until the 1960s, when the effect of the cholera toxin on fluid loss was discovered, that an effective treatment was devised: oral rehydration therapy. The whitish diarrhea produced by the toxin removed essential electrolytes. Dehydration can cause renal failure, and electrolyte loss affects signals to the heart, resulting in cardiac failure, the more common cause of death. The emetics used, lead acetate and heat applied to produce sweating, actually caused dehydration, thus increasing the likelihood of death.

Oral rehydration therapy (intravenous if necessary) is the recommended treatment today, aided by antibiotics if possible, to shorten the duration of the illness. Yet, even without antibiotics, death rates have dropped to under 1 %, an enormous decline from the 50 % and above of earlier years. The World Health Organization and disaster medicine books advise, per litre of water, 3.5 g of sodium bicarbonate, 1.5 g of potassium chloride and 20 g of glucose or 40 g of sucrose (alternatively rice or cereal).[9] Now there is a cheap, effective treatment, in short, for a disease that for more than a century was addressed with an array of, at best, harmless but ineffective ingredients, and, at worst, harmful substances.

A cholera treatment published in *The Lancet* in 1832, for example, included a mustard emetic, bloodletting (if the emetic did not suffice and the pulse continued to sink), calomel (mercury chloride), camphor and opium; externally, camphorated mercurial ointment, with oil of turpentine rubbed into the abdomen, insides of the thighs, legs and arms; heated sandbags to the extremities and sides of the body; and mustard poultices and blisters to the pit of the stomach.[10]

Civilians back in Britain sent advice on treatment to the War Office and some to Nightingale directly. With the benefit of current medical knowledge, it's clear the following typical examples would have been ineffective, but not as harmful as many in *The Lancet*, medical books and, as related in the next chapter, Mary Seacole's.

From: Wellcome Trust, RAMC 271/3–4

Recipe for cholera medicine of proved service, from Louisa Chambers, 9 January 1855, 1 oz best ginger, 1 oz cloves, 1 oz cinnamon, 1 oz nutmeg, ½ oz cayenne pepper; care that all are genuine, pulverized to finest degree; infuse in one quart of pure cognac brandy, above proof

---

[9] Gregory R. Cottone, *Disaster Medicine* 636.

[10] J. Harrison, 'Treatment of the Malignant Cholera amongst the Soldiers of the 2nd Battalion Grenadier Guards,' *The Lancet* 18,467 (11 August 1832):597.

if possible — a magnum or double bottle necessary for this quantity; shake; after tight[ly] cork, the longer the better. Dose: one dessert spoonful in half a tumbler of (2 pint cup) of hot water, as hot as can be taken, sweetened with 4 lumps white sugar. Place patient in bed between hot blankets and with hot water bottles to feet; within an hour profuse general perspiration will ensue.

Recipe from Lord Ponsonby, 1832: Place patient in bed not overloaded with clothes, 1/6 part camphor, dissolved in 6 parts of strong spirits of wine; 2 drops on a little pounded sugar in a teaspoonful of cold or iced water; five minutes later 2 more drops; continue until symptoms begin to yield. If vomiting violent, give ice before; proceed till a sense of returning warmth, perspiration and 'a manifest decrease of sickness and cramps.'

Recipe for diarrhea from Louisa Neill, 24 January 1855: half a teacupful of warmed new milk; pour into it an equal quantity of cold lime water; add 20 or 30 drops of laudanum three to six times per day; laudanum may be increased or decreased in quantity as the case requires; lime water prepared by pouring water over unshaked lime.

Recipe for diarrhea from Ean Pettis, obtained when travelling in the United States, 24 January 1855: small teacup of flour mixed with best brandy, a small quantity of lump sugar, mix to a thin paste.

Cure for diarrhea or dysentery said to be used in India: lump sugar pounded very fine; wet with the best olive oil to the consistency of a thick paste; a teaspoonful to be given three times a day.//

The official report on the Crimean War by the director general of the Army Medical Department includes a substantial chapter on cholera, drawing on numerous reports by regimental doctors. Clearly both mercury chloride (calomel) and lead acetate (sugar of lead) were used by army doctors, but there are some noteworthy sceptical reports and no claims of success. For example, on the use of 'calomel in large doses or small doses at frequent intervals,' nearly every remedy that has been recommended was tried, without success. In no case where the person recovered could any 'plan of treatment' be said to have been any more advantageous than another.[11]

In treating diarrhea in Bulgaria before the fighting began, doctors tried 'calomel, opium, mineral acids, creosote, aromatics and astringents,' but it was impossible to state any 'degree of success' (2:63). Another report described the 'terrible mortality' and 'futility of treatment' from 'various remedies' resorted 'to arrest its deadly march.' This included 'calomel, opium, mineral acids, turpentine, quinine, chloroform, arsenic, hydrocyanic [Prussic] acid, acetate of lead, stimulants [alcohol], etc.,' with fomentations, friction and heat applied externally. Further, not only were the 'resources of medicine' of 'little avail,' there was worry as to how the body, if the patient recovered, disposed of all that chloroform, arsenic, mercury chloride, opium, Prussic acid and acetate of lead (2:64).

Pathologist Robert D. Lyons conducted post-mortems on cholera victims, but found that 'the most profound and minute post-mortem researches' did not serve 'to advance our acquaintance with the *essential* nature of this ruthless plague' (2:71).

It is likely that cholera victims, as sufferers of other bowel diseases, were better off with no treatment at all. A study comparing outcomes in a cholera epidemic just before the Crimean War found that the survival rate was higher at the London Homeopathic Hospital than in the regular hospitals, 84 % to 47 %. Homeopaths had not discovered effective treatments, but used less harmful substances than regular doctors.[12]

---

[11] Cited by Andrew Smith, *Medical and Surgical History of the British Army which served in Turkey and the Crimea* 2:61.

[12] Simon Singh and Edzard Ernst, *Trick or Treatment: Alternative Medicine on Trial* 133.

The Russians

Periodically a white flag was raised and the enemies exchanged wounded soldiers and prisoners and collected their dead. The Geneva Convention on the treatment of prisoners did not exist then, but Lord Raglan believed that any Russian prisoners should get the same treatment as his own soldiers. The Russians scarcely had any opportunity to take allied prisoners; in the early battles they retreated when the allies won ground and in the later ones they were behind their fortified walls at Sebastopol, the allies outside.

The last (failed) assault made by the British Army was at the fortified bastion, the Redan, before dawn on 8 September 1855. By then the Russians had been battered by days of bombardment, which had largely destroyed the city, and had lost large numbers to desertion. Those left walked out in the night of 8–9 September after sinking their ships and setting the city on fire. There are many reminiscences of that first glimpse inside Sebastopol and awareness that the city was theirs. Astley recounted that there were 'some terrible sights in the town,' while

> in the hospital, computed to hold two thousand men, the dead were still lying in their beds, and some of the wounded who had crawled out — probably in search of food or water — had died on the floor. One of our sergeants, who had been taken prisoner a few days previously and who had been wounded, was found dead amongst a number of defunct and dying 'Ruskies.'[13]

The memoir excerpted next ends with a quotation from *Sebastopol Sketches*, the journal articles written by Leo Tolstoy, then an artillery officer at Sebastopol. He later used ideas and characters from these sketches in his famous novel *War and Peace*.

From: W. Baring Pemberton, *Battles of the Crimean War* 226–27

It will never be known who was the first to step across its shattered fortifications into a silent deserted Redan. Some time before dawn, an

---

[13] John Dugdale Astley, *Fifty Years of my Life in the World of Sport* 147.

NCO of the Royal Engineers is said to have reported it to be empty. Robert Lindsay [VC, later a founder of the British Red Cross], leading a burying party at 5 a.m., may, as he believed, have been the first to enter. Within, nothing was to be heard but the 'painful breathing and moans of the wounded who lay there amongst the dead. There were no living creatures besides the poor shattered soldiers.'...

As daylight came and the smoke cleared, the bridge of boats over which the Russians had retreated was seen to be destroyed. With this final retreat, Tolstoy closes his *Sebastopol* in words of unforgettable pathos:

On reaching the north side and on leaving the bridge almost every man took off his cap and crossed himself. But behind this feeling was another, a sad, gnawing and deeper feeling which seemed like remorse, shame and anger. Almost every soldier, looking back from the north side of the abandoned town, sighed with inexpressible bitterness in his heart and menaced the enemy.

For almost exactly a year the Russians — 'What plucky troops they were,' ejaculated the future General Gordon — had put forth a defence which evoked the admiration not only of their enemies but of the whole world. And now they were gone, with dignity and with honour, having tended our wounded as they lay in the Redan and put water within their reach.//

The Victoria Cross, awarded 'for valour,' was created at the end of the Crimean War. The medals are said still to be cast from the bronze of Russian guns captured at Sebastopol.

The Sanitary and Supply Commissions

No fewer than five commissions of investigation conducted inquiries in the East on the condition of the army and its hospitals and others took evidence in London. The commissioners of the first investigation, Cumming and Maxwell, were on the same ship as Nightingale and her nurses. Two other commissions were especially important for their mandate was to take action as well as to investigate: the Sanitary Commission under Dr John Sutherland and the Supply Commission of Sir John McNeill and Alexander Tulloch. In March 1855, the day before those commissioners arrived at Scutari, the House of Commons committee, or Roebuck committee after its chair, John Arthur Roebuck, MP, began to hold hearings in London. Nightingale would quote extensively from the evidence it collected in her *Notes on the Health of the British Army*. While the Sanitary and Supply Commissions were the two that got things done, Roebuck was the best source for who knew what and when, and who acted, or did not, on the crucial information.

Not surprisingly, the Sanitary Commission criticized lax sanitary standards and the Supply Commission inadequate supplies. Drastic changes in both areas were needed to reduce the death rates. Since both commissions started their work at the same time, it is impossible to ascertain which commission had what effect in saving lives. Nightingale initially gave more credit to the McNeill-Tulloch Commission, which improved nutrition, clothing and shelter, although she always paid attention to sanitation and ventilation. Her efforts, as can be seen in her reports and correspondence, went to address both causes of death: getting kitchens established and clothing to the soldiers as per the Supply Commission's concerns, and establishing laundries to remove excreta, vermin, etc., from bedding and clothing and removing excreta from the wards, as per the Sanitary Commission's mandate.

With the benefit of hindsight, it seems that the Sanitary Commission reforms were more crucial. Certainly Sutherland, who gave advice on nutrition to the Supply Commission, did not think that the terrible deficiencies in food, clothing and shelter were the most significant causes of the high mortality, as will be seen in his evidence below.

Given the importance of the work of the Sanitary Commission in bringing down the death rates, it is important to recognize who initiated it and with what mandate. It was not the War Office but the prime minister, Lord Palmerston, a Nightingale neighbour in Hampshire. He had been influenced by his relative by marriage Lord Shaftesbury, who had argued in the House of Lords for sanitary reforms. Palmerston's letter was delivered by Dr Sutherland, head of the commission and later the writer of its report. Sutherland was also the member to stay the longest in the East to follow through on implementation. After the war, he continued to work on sanitary reforms as a member of the Royal Commission on the Crimean War and later as the leading member of the War Office's Army Sanitary Commission, whose mandate was to ensure hygienic conditions in peacetime barracks and hospitals. He also became Nightingale's closest collaborator on nursing and hospital issues — the two worked together postwar until his retirement from illness in 1888.

From: Lord Palmerston letter to Lord Raglan, in Evelyn Ashley, *The Life and Correspondence of Henry John Temple Viscount Palmerston* 2:308–09

Downing St.

22 February 1855

This will be given to you by Dr Sutherland, chief of the Sanitary Commission, consisting of himself, Dr Gavin[14] and Mr Rawlinson, whom we have sent out to put the hospitals, the port and the camp into a less unhealthy condition than has hitherto existed, and I request that you will give them every assistance and support in your power. They will, of course, be opposed and thwarted by the medical officers, by the men who have charge of the port arrangements and by those who have the cleaning of the camp. Their mission will be ridiculed and their recommendations and directions set aside, unless enforced by the peremptory exercise of your authority.

But that authority I must request you to exert in the most peremptory manner for the immediate and exact carrying in to execution whatever changes of arrangement they may recommend, for these are matters on which depend the health and lives of many hundreds of men, I may indeed say of thousands. It is scarcely to be expected that officers,

---

[14] Hector Gavin was the doctor who suggested the Sanitary Commission to Lord Shaftesbury and then, at his request, drew up instructions for it (Georgina Battiscombe, *Shaftesbury: A Biography of the Seventh Earl* 247). He, however, was killed in a gun accident soon after arrival and was replaced by a Dr Milroy.

whether military or medical, whose time is wholly occupied by the pressing business of each day, should be able to give their attention or their time to the matters to which these commissioners have for many years devoted their action and their thoughts.

But the interposition of men skilled in this way is urgently required. The hospital at Scutari is become a hotbed of pestilence, and if no proper precautions are taken before the sun's rays begin to be felt, your camp will become one vast seat of the most virulent plague. I hope this commission will arrive in time to prevent much evil, but I am very sure that not one hour should be lost after their arrival in carrying into effect the precautionary and remedial measures which they may recommend.//

Lord Panmure's four-page letter to the commission is also worth quoting. It instructed them to depart with 'utmost expedition' (in fact they left within three days) and to ensure that they obtained 'full powers' from the various commanders to get into every hospital and camp, insisting 'no time is to be lost,' and that they were to remove, 'as far as is possible, all evil influences' in the air. They were to inspect and then state what should be done in 'cleansing, disinfecting or of actual construction' for safety and health, as 'speedily as possible.'

The commission members were not to rest content with an order, but to 'see instantly, by yourselves or by your agents, to the commencement of the work, and to its superintendence day by day until it is finished,' a point Dr Sutherland took to heart. The camp, also, was to come to their 'immediate and anxious attention,' to ensure that the 'best antidotes or preventives to the deadly exhalations' would be used against the emissions 'from the saturated soil whenever the warmth of spring shall begin to act on the surface.'[15]

Several excerpts will be given from the report of the Sanitary Commission, but we begin with one excerpt from that of the Supply

---

[15] Panmure letter to the commissioners, in Sutherland, *Report of the Sanitary Commission* 1–2.

Commission. The effectiveness of their combined efforts will be revisited at the end of this chapter with data comparing British and French Army death rates.

From: UK, *Report of the Commission of Inquiry into the Supplies of the British Army in the Crimea*, First Report, 10 June 1855 1–3, 8

We ascertained that the sick arriving from the Crimea were nearly all suffering from diseases chiefly attributable to diet, and that the food supplied to the army during the winter, consisting principally of salt meat and biscuit, with a very insufficient proportion of vegetables, was calculated, in the circumstances in which the troops were placed, to produce those diseases....

It was inevitable that the operations of a siege carried on throughout the winter in the Crimea should involve a very considerable amount of hardship and sickness....The sickness and consequent mortality in the British Army in the Crimea have, however, been very great. The deaths, including those at Scutari and elsewhere, appear to amount to about 35 percent of the average strength of the army present in the Crimea from the 1st of October 1854 to the 30th of April 1855, and it seems to be clearly established that this excessive mortality is not to be attributed to anything peculiarly unfavourable in the climate, but to overwork, exposure to wet and cold, improper food, insufficient clothing during part of the winter, and insufficient shelter from inclement weather.

The health of the army also suffered from a deficiency of fresh or preserved vegetables. Lord Raglan seems to have been urged to supply the deficiency, but it appears that, according to the Regulations, vegetables do not constitute a part of the soldier's rations, and it is, therefore, no part of the ordinary duty of the Commissariat to issue or even to provide them. This arrangement, which leaves the soldier to purchase vegetables in the market, may be an advantage to him where such a market exists, but it is obviously inapplicable where, as in the Crimea, there was none. The first attempts to import green vegetables were not successful, and some time elapsed before the defects in the arrangements could be so far remedied as to secure a regular supply. In the meantime, scurvy in its ordinary form, and scorbutic diseases in various forms, extended rapidly til, in several regiments, hardly a man was free from the taint.//

The Report of the Sanitary Commission, 301 pages, is a key document for understanding what went wrong in the war hospitals, camps and the town of Balaclava, what measures were taken to reduce death rates from sanitary defects and the process of getting the work done and checked. It influenced the work of the later Royal Commission, of which Sutherland was a member, and to which both he and Nightingale gave evidence. The report is a model of applied research, one that Nightingale, as it will be seen in Chapter 4, followed in her own work after the war and indeed for the rest of her working life. The commission was composed of top experts in the field of sanitation, headed by Dr Sutherland, who had been the first public health officer in the UK, in Liverpool, the city which pioneered sanitary reform, with two experienced sanitary experts, James Newlands, the first borough engineer in England, and James Wilson, inspector of nuisances. The diary notes of both these men give precise details on the amounts of filth and dead animals removed from the hospitals and camps, which Sutherland incorporated into his official report. The other significant commissioner was Robert Rawlinson, a civil engineer and leading water expert (later, like Dr Sutherland, a close collaborator of Nightingale).

The report set out the sanitary problems hospital by hospital, with the gory details of sewers, drains and filth. It detailed the inspections to be conducted to ascertain the work had been properly done and that the rebuilding actually worked. Interspersed were statistics on hospital admissions and deaths to show that reductions occurred after the clean-up. There were precise recommendations for future application.

Sutherland's analysis on death rates by hospital would reappear in quotations in Nightingale's longer and more comprehensive report. Clearly the two saw eye to eye and probably discussed their findings in the course of their respective writing.

His report began with the Barrack Hospital at Scutari, the largest hospital and the first inspected, beginning the day the commission arrived. Its 'open and airy' site was about the only thing to be commended, a point Nightingale herself would often make. His report continues: 'On entering the hospital, the first thing that attracted our attention was the defective state of the ventilation.' Except for a few small openings, there were 'no means of renewing the atmosphere within the hospital' (11–12). Both wards and corridors were occupied, so that it was like two hospitals built back to back, 'with the foul air in each intermingling by the doors....The sewers and drains were badly formed, badly constructed, badly laid and untrapped' (12). Bedpans containing excreta were left in the wards (14). The cleansing operations included the outskirts, the removal of dead animals, opening and flushing out the sewers, and evacuating and closing wards. The graveyard was disinfected and new rules instituted for burials (13).

Yet, bad as the sanitary defects at the Barrack Hospital were, they were worse at the hospital at Koulali, which had the highest death rates in the war and was not under Nightingale's administration. Dr Sutherland's commission found the only positive feature of the Koulali hospital was its convenient location for disembarking patients (23). The sanitary defects began with the privies, whose emanations 'pervaded' the building. The ventilation was 'very imperfect and the wards overcrowded' (24). The commission directed substantial rebuilding, but even then, it will be seen, Koulali remained a relatively unhealthy hospital.

A table in the report gave the death rates per sick cases after the drastic renovations had been completed, showing the Barrack Hospital improving to the lowest rate of the four at 1.8 % deaths to sick cases (63). Sutherland also compared death rates at these four main Bosphorus hospitals beginning before the commission's arrival. Again the percentages of deaths per sick cases declined as follows:

Barrack Hospital, from 7.5 % to 1.1 %
General Hospital, from 11.7 % to 1.3 %
Palace Hospital, from 7.4 % to 0.8 %
Koulali Hospital, from 11.3 % to 0.7 % (50).

The Koulali decline is noticeably the largest, a point Sutherland would make in his evidence to the Royal Commission.

The great superiority, in sanitary matters, of the Crimea hospitals over those of the Bosphorus, quickly became apparent:

> The Castle Hospital was situated on one of the finest natural positions that could have been selected for such a purpose. It occupied the whole of a long narrow ridge running nearly east and west....The natural means of drainage were all that could have been desired, and the esplanade towards the sea was always dry.

The huts faced the sea, and water came from a spring-fed well (133).

The report, as the next extract shows, had only praise for the new pre-fabricated hut hospital at Renkioi, about 100 miles from Scutari. Designed by engineer I.K. Brunel, it had state-of-the-art toilet and washing arrangements. No renovations were needed. As well, the site had been deliberately chosen for its advantages: high ground sloping to the sea, easy landing and a clean water supply.

From: John Sutherland, *Report of the Sanitary Commission* 59

> The wards [at Renkioi] were large, lofty, wooden huts, many times more capacious than any in the Crimea, arranged so as to form three lanes perpendicular to the sea, ensuring thereby a free sweep of the sea breeze among the huts....
>
> Each ward had eight water closets, with urinals and lavatories, all abundantly supplied with water, and outside the ward. There can be no question that this hospital offered great sanitary advantages for the recovery of the sick. The situation is one of the best the country affords. The wards were clean, lofty and admitted of any amount of ventilation. There was abundance of space for the sick.//

However, as a later book on Renkioi Hospital pointed out, any comparison between it and the Scutari hospitals should only be made for the period that both were open. For those dates, from October 1855 to June 1856, the death rate was 4.7 % at Scutari and 3.8 % at Renkioi,[16] a difference to be sure but far less than 'double' as some findings claimed.

Sir John Hall challenged key findings of the *Report of the Sanitary Commission*, arguing that the Army Medical Department had done all that was necessary.[17] Sutherland rebutted him in evidence he subsequently gave to the Royal Commission, as provided below. The term 'zymotic' which appears was used, when specific disease bacilli were not known, for epidemic diseases, especially typhus and typhoid fever, scarlet fever and cholera.

From: John Sutherland, Evidence 17 July 1857, UK, *Report of the Commissioners [on...] the Sanitary Condition of the Army and the Treatment of the Sick and Wounded* 2:334

The great hospitals at Scutari were magnificent buildings, apparently admirably adapted for their purpose when superficially looked at, but, when carefully examined, they were found to be little better than pest houses. The drainage of all the hospitals was in the highest degree defective and dangerous; the sewers were untrapped and unventilated; they were loaded with filth to such an extent that, during the first week of our sanitary works, no less than 100 hand carts of filth were removed from the sewers of the Barrack and General Hospitals. These immense sewer cesspools communicated with the interior of the hospitals by a large number of open pipes to the privies, and, in certain states of the wind, sewer air was blown over this mass of filth directly into the atmosphere of the wards and corridors, for none of these sewers and privies had any other means of ventilation at that time except into the hospitals, and fever among the sick and healthy was the result.

At Koulali, where the sanitary defects were even more serious, there were fifty open privies and 200 cavalry horses under wards and

---

[16] Christopher Silver, *Renkioi: Brunel's Forgotten Crimean War Hospital* 120.

[17] John Hall, *Observations on the Report of the Sanitary Commissioners in the Crimea, During the Years 1855 and 1856.*

quarters, and fatal cases of fever had arisen directly traceable to these causes. No sufficient means of ventilation had been provided in any of these hospitals....

There was an overcharged burial ground close to the walls of the General Hospital. It will be evident, at a glance, that to place either sick or healthy people in any number in these buildings was to endanger health and life; even healthy people died in them from zymotic diseases; how much more likely to suffer were men in so susceptible a state of constitution as were those who came from the Crimea to Scutari at the beginning of 1855, and yet we are expected to overlook the obvious consequences of such neglects, and to seek for the causes of the enormous mortality in the Crimea....

It is hardly possible to conceive any more striking sanitary contrast than those hospitals presented before and after these measures were put in force....Within the first three weeks of the improvements the mortality in all the hospitals fell to one half of what it was during the three weeks before. In three weeks more it was down to one third. During the next three weeks it had fallen to less than a fourth, and in six weeks more it was less than a tenth. At Koulali the mortality fell to an 18th part of what it was when the sanitary works were commenced, but at that hospital the defects were the most serious, and the loss of life from them had been the greatest.//

British Army superiority to the French Army

The great success of the Sanitary and Supply Commissions can be seen in the marked differences in death rates between the British and French Armies in the first and second winters of the war. Thanks to the Sanitary and Supply Commissions, British soldiers had far better food, clothing and shelter in the second winter, and camp and hospital hygiene was vastly improved. The French did nothing comparable, and their lower death rates (they arrived better prepared) went up terribly in the second year. Firm data for the French were not available until seven years after the war, but the fact of their worsening death rates was well known. Sutherland assessed it as follows:

> During the same period of 1856, when the British troops in the Crimea were in a better sanitary condition and more healthy than they are in barracks at home, the French Army before Sebastopol was decimated by typhus and other zymotic maladies chiefly connected with the defective sanitary state of most of their camps, and the overcrowded, unventilated and unwholesome condition of tents, huts, hospitals and transports.[18]

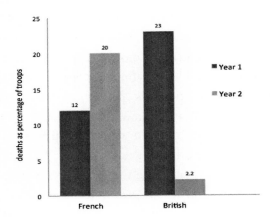

When the French data became available, the differences were staggering. They show that the British reduced their death rate from 23 % in the first winter to 2.2 % in the second, while the French rate rose from 12 % to a colossal 20 %[19] even when hostilities were over and there were no casualties from battle. This demonstrates unequivocally the effectiveness of the Sanitary and Supply Commissions, a conclusion shared by French doctors in their later assessments. Léon Le Fort, for example, argued that French war hospitals were inferior to both the British and Russian

---

[18] Sutherland, *Report of the Sanitary Commission* 193.

[19] Jean-Charles Chenu, *De la mortalité dans l'armée et moyens d'économiser le vie humaine* 131.

versions[20] and flagged the role of Nightingale and the commissions sent out as crucial.[21] Baudens judged the British war hospitals to have been cleaner and the food better, thanks to the greater power of their army doctors to implement improvements.[22] He also noted that the British considered soldiers as 'capital' and treated them better (630).

The British Army continued to apply the lessons of the Crimean War at home, so that death rates in barracks and army hospitals back in the UK fell after the war. The French did not, nor did they make improvements before the next serious war, the Franco-Prussian War of 1870–71. Credit for Britain's post-war reforms belongs to Nightingale and the Army Sanitary Commission, which was set up precisely to act on the Royal Commission recommendations for reform.

The Crimean War produced many heroes. If there is an 'unsung hero' to celebrate, my vote would go to Dr Sutherland as the person who most deserves credit for drastically reducing the British Army's death rates in the second half of the war. After the war, he continued to be a civilian employee of the War Office but worked in effect as Nightingale's research assistant and often as editor, as they jointly took up the challenge of health care and hospital reform in civil society.

---

[20] Léon Le Fort, 'Le service de santé dans les armées nouvelles: Observations et souvenirs de la dernière guerre,' *Revue des deux mondes* 96 (1 November 1871):88.

[21] Le Fort, 'La campagne d'Italie en 1859,' *Oeuvres de Léon Le Fort* 3:57.

[22] L. Baudens, 'Une mission médicale à l'Armée d'Orient. III. Les hôpitaux, les Épidémies et le typhus de Crimée, dernière partie,' *Revue des deux mondes* (1 June 1857):594.

Chapter 3

The wonderful adventures of Mrs Seacole

Birth, childhood, travels, marriage

Mary Seacole, as she will be referred to here, was born Mary Jane Grant in Kingston, Jamaica. The date of her birth is uncertain (no registry or baptismal records are available). The ages she gave on the 1871 and 1881 UK censuses were sixty and seventy, respectively, which would have her born in 1811. However, her death certificate in 1881 gave her age as seventy-six and thus 1805 is usually given as her year of birth. She was raised by her mother, a lodging house keeper who was also an 'admirable doctress,' or herbalist. Her mother was of mixed-race. Her 'soldier' father was white and presumably in the British Army, but she gave no further details about him, not even his name, date of death or details of his departure — he simply disappears from the memoir on page 1. Seacole herself was probably three-quarters white and lived in a white world. Her memoir states: 'I am a Creole, and have good Scotch blood coursing in my veins' (1). She distanced herself from those Creole (she never said African) roots: 'I am only a little brown — a few shades duskier than the brunettes whom you all admire so much' (4). She attributed her industry to her Scotch heritage: 'I have often heard the term "lazy Creole" applied to my country people, but I am sure I do not know what it is to be indolent' (2).

Seacole was placed for some years (exactly when is not specified) with 'an old lady who brought me up in her household among her own grandchildren' (2). It is not known if she was given any formal education (she mentioned none), but her mother instructed her in traditional Creole remedies. She learned much by assisting when 'invalid officers or their wives' came to the boarding house from the army stations at Up-Park or Newcastle. She had, as a girl, a 'yearning for medical knowledge and practice' (2).

The Grants were free, middle-class property owners at a time when slavery still existed in Jamaica — it was not fully abolished until 1838. Neither Seacole, nor her family, were poor or working class, but neither did they belong to the white elite. Like white Jamaicans, they employed blacks. It seems that, on her mother's death, Seacole inherited her boarding house, Blundell Hall, although it is not named in the memoir nor any details given of her taking charge of it. The National Library of Jamaica now occupies the site and a plaque recognizes it as Seacole's former home.

On her Panama travels and in the Crimea, Seacole was accompanied by her black maid, Mary (39, 57), and another black servant, Mac (12). At her store in the Crimea she employed two black cooks in addition to them. In Panama, she was called the 'yellow woman from Jamaica' (27) and the 'yellow doctress' (34), evidently acceptable terms to her, indicating her light skin. She referred to herself as a 'motherly yellow woman' in 1854 (78) when she formed the idea of going to the Crimean War. She never described herself as black.

Seacole made two trips to England when young — no dates are given. On the second, she stayed two years, earning her living by selling 'a large stock of West Indian preserves and pickles' (4). She next traveled to New Providence (in the Bahamas), Haiti and Cuba, acquiring 'handsome shells and rare shellwork' in the Bahamas to sell back in Jamaica, where they caused 'quite a sensation' (5). She then 'nursed' her old patroness in her dying days (5).

She married Edwin Horatio Hamilton Seacole, a merchant, in 1836. He was a sickly man, about whom virtually nothing is known. His family called him the natural child of Admiral Horatio Nelson and his mistress, Lady Hamilton, but there is no firm evidence for this speculation. Seacole called him Nelson's godson in her will, where she left a ring Nelson was said to have given him to her benefactor, Count Gleichen. Seacole biographer Jane Robinson went to some trouble to try to track down the relationship, to no avail.[1] A similar first name may mean nothing, for people often named a child after a famous person, which the hero of the Battle of Trafalgar and conqueror of Napoleon most decidedly was.

The couple settled in Black River, where they ran a store together. She 'kept him alive by kind nursing and attention as long as I could' (5), but when he became very ill and the store failed, they returned to Kingston to her mother's house, where he died (6). For neither her husband nor her patroness did Seacole mention any specific treatments or name any disease or cause of death (5–6). Her mother died soon after (again, no dates or cause of death are given).

Seacole's 'poor home' (7), presumably Blundell Hall, burned down in 1843 — a rare mention of a specific year — in a great fire which devastated Kingston on 29 August. After rebuilding, she may have sold or given the house to her sister, or possibly the two inherited it jointly. Her sister was running Blundell Hall when Anthony Trollope stayed there in 1858–59 (his comments are quoted later in this chapter).

As in her mother's time, Seacole's guests were army and navy officers and their wives, all white, some of 'high rank' (8). Neither mother nor daughter ran a convalescent or nursing home, but both looked after their guests when they fell ill and took in ill persons, especially during major epidemics. Seacole described learning much from naval and army surgeons who stayed there (8).

In 1850 a cholera epidemic 'swept over the island of Jamaica with terrible force.' A doctor lodging at Seacole's house gave her 'many hints as to its treatment' (8–9). Early that same year, her half-brother started up a 'considerable store and hotel' in Panama (9), for men en route overland (there was no Panama Canal then) to take part in the California Gold Rush. To supply the prospectors, she had clothing and foods made for sale:

---

[1] Jane Robinson, *Mary Seacole: The Charismatic Black Nurse Who Became a Heroine of the Crimea* 30–32.

My house was full for weeks of tailors making up rough coats, trousers, etc., and sempstresses cutting out and making shirts....My kitchen was filled with busy people manufacturing preserves, guava jelly and other delicacies.

She invested 'a considerable sum' in the purchase of preserved meats, vegetables and eggs (9).

In Cruces, where her brother established his Independent Hotel, conditions were grim and the amenities few (see her Chapter 2 for the trip there, Chapter 3 for the hotel). Cholera soon arrived and there was no doctor to provide treatment. Seacole diagnosed the sick and prescribed treatments, gratis when patients could not pay (see her Chapter 4 for details). She soon opened her own store and restaurant (Chapter 5 in her memoir), which she called the 'British Hotel,' although, unlike her brother's establishment, it was not actually a hotel.

Since there was no doctor at Cruces when the epidemic broke out, Seacole was on her own dealing with the stricken. Her memoir records her belief, which she shared with 'her people' (meaning Jamaican Creoles) but not 'the faculty' (meaning medical doctors), that cholera was contagious (24). She described it first appearing in one man, a Spaniard, then quickly spreading to his friends (25). Cholera in fact is not contagious by touch but is transmitted by bacilli in fecal-laden water.

There was a dentist in Cruces, Seacole explained, but he refused to prescribe treatments, so she worked alone. A Spanish doctor in Panama was sent for, but, when he arrived, he proved to be unfamiliar with cholera and let her carry on. She described being paid 'handsomely' by some patients and receiving only thanks from others (27).

For her first (claimed) cure, she described using 'mustard emetics, warm fomentations, mustard plasters on the stomach and the back, and calomel [mercury chloride], at first in large then in gradually smaller doses' (25). Seacole noted that natives of Panama, who were especially badly hit, confronted the disease by prostrating themselves before 'tawdry dirty saints supposed to possess some miraculous influence' (26), but they would not stir a finger 'to clean out their close, reeking huts or rid the damp streets of the rotting accumulation of months' (27). She succeeded in getting a mule owner to throw open doors and shutters, light fires and ventilate the hut, but two patients 'were beyond my skill' (28). Because of the terrible groans from the sufferers, she had 'rude screens' fixed up around the dying men (29). She noted the 'daily, almost hourly, scenes of death' (30).

The last patient Seacole described tying to cure was 'a brown-faced orphan infant, scarce a year old' (29). After it died in her arms, she bribed the man who took the body away to take it to the river and let her perform a post-mortem on it, which he did. This was her 'first and last' post-mortem (30) and she considered that the knowledge she obtained from it 'very valuable' and 'soon put into practice.' As noted in the previous chapter, however, pathologist Robert D. Lyons found nothing by his dissections that shed any light on the course of the disease. It is now known that the loss of electrolytes is crucial to the loss of life and this is not discernible by autopsy.

In her work at Cruces, Seacole acknowledged making 'lamentable blunders' at first and that she 'lost patients which a little later I could have saved.' When she came across some notes of cholera medicines she had used, they made her 'shudder, and I dare say they have been used in their turn and found wanting' (31).

The simplest remedies were 'perhaps the best': mustard plasters, emetics and calomel, 'mercury applied externally.' Opium she rather dreaded, 'for it lulls the patient into a sleep,' often the 'sleep of death.' For thirst she gave 'water in which cinnamon had been boiled.' For a 'stubborn attack,' she added a 'dose of ten grains of sugar of lead [lead acetate], mixed in a pint of water given in doses of a tablespoonful every quarter of an hour' (31). She came to the conclusion that 'few constitutions permitted the use of exactly similar remedies, and that the course of treatment which saved one man would, if persisted in, have very likely killed his brother' (31–32). This is an extraordinarily frank statement, but one that does not appear in comments by Seacole campaigners. Sugar of lead, or lead acetate, as noted in the previous chapter (p 50), causes dehydration and has toxic properties.

Seacole's Panama adventures take up three chapters in her memoir and include running the business, finding supplies, hiring staff, and dealing with thieves, prisoners, fights and visiting Americans, as well as looking after the sick. She briefly ran a hotel mainly for women travelers in Gorgona, a bad experience overall (49–50).

In Chapter 6, as she prepared to leave Cruces, Seacole met with overt racism from some Americans — slavery was still the law in the American South. She handled the two encounters she recounts with verve. In the first, a man toasting her called her 'the best yaller woman' that God ever made. But he was vexed that she was not 'wholly white' and mused that 'if we could bleach her' to make her 'acceptable,' they would (47). Seacole declined the bleach job and said that, if her complexion 'had been as dark as any nigger's, I should have been just as happy and as useful.' She did not think she would lose much by being excluded from white society. She drank 'to you and the general reformation of American manners' (48). Seacole's stand was principled — for racial equality — while at the same time it distanced her from blacks. Her skin was obviously not 'as dark as any nigger's.'

Seacole faced overt racism again when she, with her black maid, were refused entry to the ladies' compartment on an American steamer returning to Kingston. Seacole went to the captain and got their fares refunded and they returned without incident on a British ship soon after (56–58).

Back in Jamaica, now in 1853, a terrible yellow fever epidemic broke out (related in her Chapter 7). Seacole described the misery of the people in her boarding house — officers, wives and children. Her treatments did not work and some people were so far gone by the time she saw them that nothing could be done to ease their suffering. She claimed not one cure at any stage of the epidemic but spared the reader much misery by limiting her description of the course of the epidemic to five pages (59–63).

In a passage normally misinterpreted or truncated, Seacole described military authorities asking her 'to provide nurses for the sick at Up-Park Camp, about a mile from Kingston' (59). This is typically understood to mean that Seacole followed through on this and even that she led a professional British Army nursing service there, a subject dealt with in Chapter 5. But her own statement shows that she did not: 'leaving some nurses and my sister at home, I went there and did my best, but it was little we could do to mitigate the severity of the epidemic' (63). Moreover, she could hardly have led a team of professional nurses at the army camp, for the British Army did not employ professional nurses at *any* camp at that time.[2] It is clear from her memoir that there were no nurses, of any description, present (63).

After the epidemic, Seacole made another trip to Panama to wind up her business and visit the town with her brother. She then ran a store for three months at Navy Bay, but the quarrels and bloodshed there and a potential native uprising made her leave (64). She next went to Escribanos, where the New Granada Gold Mining Company was in operation, 'the only portion of my life devoted to gold seeking' (65). She tried, unsuccessfully, to sell what she thought was gold (69) and described joining a prospecting trip (70–71).

It was at Escribanos that Seacole met Thomas Day, a relative of her late husband, who would later be her business partner in the Crimea — he was then superintendent of the gold mine (66). He fell ill, but she 'was able to nurse Mr Day through a sharp attack of illness' (69). What the illness was and what she did for him, she did not say.

On leaving Escribanos, Seacole stopped for a short time at Navy Bay, then went on direct to England, where she had 'claims on a mining company which are still unsatisfied' (71). Her shares in the Palmilla Mine speculation brought her to London in the autumn of 1854, shortly after the first battle of the Crimean War; the more heroic — but fictional — version is in Chapter 5 of this book.

The Crimean War

Seacole credited her soldier father with her early interest in war and her 'affection for camp life...the pomp, pride and circumstance of glorious war' (1). Postwar, in her letter to Lord Rokeby, she referred to the 'brave

---

[2] When it earlier employed nurses, they were recruited from among the wives and widows of privates and non-commissioned officers, were paid less than cooks and laundresses, and reported to a sergeant, not a doctor (Fred Smith, *A Short History of the Royal Army Medical Corps* 11–14).

defenders of our country,'[3] although the Russians were hardly about to invade England in 1854. In her letter to *Punch*, she called the Crimean War 'a noble contest.'[4] Her interest in what became the Crimean War was aroused while still in Jamaica, before the Escribanos trip, by the departure of regiments for the East, which began in roughly March 1854. She explained, 'no sooner had I heard of war somewhere than I longed to witness it' (73). However, she did not follow the regiments but went on to Navy Bay on her gold mining venture.

Her memoir tells us that Seacole arrived in London to attend to her gold speculation 'just after the battle of Alma had been fought' (74), which was on 20 September 1854. She described longing 'more than ever' to suffer 'for a cause it was so glorious to fight and bleed for!' (75–76). Newspaper advertisements for hospital nurses were published, but Seacole did not apply (the applications are housed at the National Archives, Kew). When Nightingale and her nurses left England for the war on 21 October 1854, Seacole was still pursuing her gold mining investments. It was only after the sinking of a supply ship, the *Prince*, on 14 November 1854, that she found herself increasingly inclined 'to join my old friends of the 97th, 48th and other regiments,' so she 'threw over the gold speculation altogether and devoted all my energies to my new scheme' (74). She confided a desire to become 'a Crimean *heroine*' (76).

On the day that Nightingale and her team departed for the war, Sidney Herbert, secretary at war, the junior war minister, wrote an official letter on nursing, which was widely published. In it he stated that Nightingale and her nurses had departed for the war and that no further nurses would be sent until and unless she explicitly asked for them (in fact the next lot were sent without her requesting them or the doctors wanting them). His letter explained that a register of applicants was being kept and gave three addresses where people might leave their names, one of which was his

---

[3] 'Mrs Seacole,' *The Times* 29 November 1856 12D.

[4] 'Our Own Vivandière,' *Punch* 30 May 1857 p. 221.

home at Belgrave Square. Applicants who lacked hospital experience were directed to the third name, Mrs Gipps, at St John's Hospital (properly, St John's House), Queen Square.[5]

Seacole did not say exactly when she decided she wanted to go to the war, only that it was after the sinking of the supply ship, the *Prince*, which occurred on 14 November. However, news of that disaster (the ship carried winter clothing and medical supplies) did not reach London until the end of the month.[6] By then the second contingent of nurses was well along getting the required hospital experience and otherwise preparing for departure. That group consisted of Irish Sisters of Mercy from several convents, as well as other 'ladies' and ordinary hospital nurses — a number larger than Nightingale's original thirty-eight. The Sisters of Mercy left Ireland for London on 3 November,[7] and their leader, Mary Francis Bridgeman, who was the superior of the convent at Kinsale, met with the leader of the full group, Mary Stanley, on 12 November. They spent several weeks at London hospitals for basic training, leaving for the East on 2 December 1854 (125).

Instead of applying in the prescribed manner, Seacole went directly to the War Office, which did not interview or hire nurses. She tried unsuccessfully to get an interview with the secretary at war, but he did not interview or hire either, nor did the quartermaster general, whose offices she next visited (*WA* 76–77). A gentleman at that office recommended that she go to the Army Medical Department (78) which officially did the hiring, although they did not interview or select. She found the private address of the secretary at war and went there (78). Seacole was again disappointed and suspected that 'American prejudices against colour' were to blame for her not being accepted to go out with the second lot (79). Whether or not racism was a factor, we do not know: she was old

---

[5] Sidney Herbert letter to Nightingale of 21 October, published as 'Nurses for the Wounded,' *The Times* 24 October 1854 9A.

[6] 'The Gale in the Black Sea,' *The Times* 30 November 1854 7A.

[7] Maria Luddy, ed., *The Crimean Journals of the Sisters of Mercy 1854–56* 8.

for a nurse, nearing fifty (retirement was typically at sixty), lacked the formal training and hospital experience demanded, and missed the brief hospital training provided to others who lacked experience. Preparations for the second group's departure were well along before she even contemplated trying to join.

While all this was going on, Seacole ran into Thomas Day, who was on his way to Balaclava on shipping business. They 'came to the understanding that (if it were found desirable) we should together open a store as well as a hotel in the neighbourhood of the camp,' thus forming the business of 'Seacole and Day' (81).

Seacole announced her plan to establish the 'British Hotel' by sending printed cards to her 'former kind friends and to the officers of the Army and Navy generally.' She described the venture as 'a mess table and comfortable quarters for sick and convalescent officers' (81), or 'a hotel for invalids' (80). Her 'limited capital' was sufficient to purchase supplies, including unspecified 'home comforts' and medicines (81–82). She did not have to borrow money to make the trip, as is often suggested. The printed card gave her expected departure from London as 25 January 1855 on the *Hollander*.[8] The official report of the Army Medical Department, which sent medical supplies on the same ship, gave the departure date as 10 February 1855, with arrival at Scutari on 8 March 1855.[9]

Seacole's Chapter 8 relates the (above) efforts in London to get to the war. Chapter 9 relates the journey, and her one, brief meeting with Nightingale, at Scutari. Seacole describes walking through the wards, greeting soldiers who recognized her from Jamaica (87–89). Late in the day, she sought a bed for the night as she was leaving for Balaclava the next morning. She spoke with Mrs Bracebridge (89), who was assisting Nightingale at the hospital, and then with Nightingale herself, whom she

---

[8] Robinson gave a departure date of 27 January, in *Mary Seacole* 91; Orlando Figes gave a departure, from Gravesend, ship unspecified, on 15 February 1855, in *Crimea: The Last Crusade* 354.

[9] Smith, *Medical and Surgical History of the British Army* 1:532.

described as 'a slight figure, in the nurses' dress, with a pale, gentle and withal firm face' (90). She gave Nightingale a letter from a Dr F., whom she had met in Malta en route but knew from Jamaica (85). Nightingale read it and asked what she could do for her: 'If it lies in my power, I shall be very happy' (91). Seacole asked for and was given a bed for the night and breakfast was taken to her in the morning (92). She then proceeded to her ship to travel to Balaclava. Chapters 10–12 describe the nitty gritty of setting up her huts, with all the problems of getting in supplies and dealing with unreliable employees and thieves.

Alexis Soyer, the chef who volunteered to establish kitchens and improve nutrition for the troops, was an early visitor. An officer introduced them:

> God bless you, my son, are you Monsieur Soyer of whom I heard so much in Jamaica? Well, to be sure! I have sold many and many a score of your relish and other sauces — God knows how many.

She promptly invited him to 'take a glass of champagne with my old friend, Sir John Campbell.' Soyer, as the next extract shows, convinced Seacole not to provide for overnight stays, but to keep her business focused on food and drink.[10] The two got along well. He complimented her on her soups and dainties (*WA* 149) and she called him 'my son.'

From: Alexis Soyer, *Culinary Campaign* 233

> The old lady expressed her desire to consult me about what she should do to make money in her new speculation, in which she had embarked a large capital, pointing to two iron houses in course of construction on the other side of the road. She told me that her intention was to have beds there for visitors, which I persuaded her not to do, saying 'all the visitors — and they are few in number — sleep on board the vessels in the harbour, and the officers under canvass in the camp. Lay in a good stock of hams, wines, spirits, ale and porter, sauces, pickles and a few

---

[10] Soyer, *Culinary Campaign* 231–32.

preserves and dry vegetables — in short anything which will not spoil by keeping.' 'Yes,' said she, 'I mean to have all that.'//

Because of delays in the arrival of supplies, Seacole spent her first six weeks organizing on shore by day, but sleeping on a boat by night (96). She recounted that, during this time, she helped doctors transfer the sick and wounded into the transports to take them to the general hospitals. The scenes on that 'fearful wharf' were 'heartrending' (98). The death rate during those transports was also fearful, much discussed in Nightingale's and official army reports. Seacole described bringing sponge cake, tea and lemonade, 'all the doctors would allow me to give to the wounded' (101).

The next extract is from a late memoir (published in 1911) of an army doctor who met Seacole at the wharf when he accompanied an officer to a boat for embarkation.

From: Douglas Arthur Reid, *Memories of the Crimean War* 13–14

On reaching Balaclava we were directed to the wooden landing stage, where boats were ready to take the sick and wounded to the hospital ships. Here I made the acquaintance of a celebrated person, Mrs Seacole, a coloured woman, who, out of the goodness of her heart and at her own expense, supplied hot tea to the poor sufferers while they were waiting to be lifted into the boats. I need not say how grateful they were for the warm and comforting beverage when they were benumbed with cold and exhausted by the long and trying journey from the front. The temperature was many degrees below freezing point....

A few words more about Mrs Seacole. She did not spare herself if she could do any good to the suffering soldiers. In rain and snow, in storm and tempest, day after day she was at her self-chosen post, with her stove and kettle, in any shelter she could find, brewing tea for all who wanted it, and they were many. Sometimes more than 200 sick would be embarked in one day, but Mrs Seacole was always equal to the occasion.//

Seacole gave no date for the opening of their enterprise, but said that by summer, though not finished, it was at least well in operation (113). The main hut consisted of a long iron room with counters and a little kitchen. There were two small huts with sleeping rooms for herself and her business partner, outhouses for the servants, 'a canteen for the soldiery' (114) and an enclosed yard for horses, mules, sheep, goats, geese and fowl (117). It was never a hotel or hospital. The memoir goes into considerable detail as to the goods that could be purchased and the meals served (Chapters 12, 14 and 18).

Seacole had no way of knowing this, but when she arrived in the East in March 1855, war hospital death rates had started to decline and conditions in the camp were improving: the worst month for deaths was January (3168), while February had 2523 (both are slight underestimates, as some categories were omitted).[11] Deaths dropped substantially in March (1409), the month that the Sanitary and Supply Commissions began their work. Also in March 1855, the railway to connect the port with the camps became operational, which vastly improved the arrival of supplies and reduced the workload of the men who previously had to haul them.

Chapter 13 includes numerous excerpts from letters purportedly sent to Mrs Seacole by satisfied patients, most of them unnamed. It also has letters purportedly written by senior army officers, on which more will be said later.

Chapter 14 cheerfully relates the food available for purchase at the store: tins of salmon, lobsters, oysters, sardines, game, wild fowl, vegetables, eggs, and a good joint of mutton, plus such items as tobacco, snuff, cigarette papers and saddlery (139). In hot weather, there were claret and cider cups, sangria and other cooling drinks (151). At Christmas she made plum puddings (recipe provided) and mince pies for dinner parties (185–86). On New Year's Day she took a batch of plum puddings and mince pies to the nearby Land Transport Corps hospital (187) as a gift.

---

[11] Smith, *Medical and Surgical History of the British Army* vol. 2, Table A.

Wonderful Adventures records visits by distinguished people, including a French prince, duke and viscount (178–80). Seacole visited the 'Turkish pasha' and formed a 'lasting friendship' with him (110). He drank her bottled beer, sherry and champagne (114). He became a frequent visitor — Seacole describes giving him English lessons, for which she claims no success (111). She never met Lord Raglan but did see him riding through camp on horseback. When he was dying, she got his servants to let her have a 'peep into the room' where he lay (161). She attended his funeral 'turned out with the brightest of ribbons in her bonnet,' as a memoir of the time described her.[12]

Most of the testimonials to her work published in her memoir do not include full names or adequate identifying information (127–32). However, two senior officers given only initials can be easily identified:

* 'Wm P–, adjutant general of the British Army in the Crimea,' could only be Lord William Paulet, who is quoted as praising her for 'attending wounded men, even in positions of great danger';
* 'C.A.W–, Lt-Gen, Comm. of Sebastopol' could only be General Sir Charles Ash Windham, who is quoted saying that she was 'a useful and good person, kind and charitable' (132).

Two officers killed at the Redan, whom she called friends, are identified with initials only:

* 'Sir John C–,' a 'kind patron for years' (159), must be John Campbell, second baronet, to whom she was serving champagne when Soyer dropped by. Campbell had served in the West Indies, among many places; he died at the Redan after rashly leading his men in battle;
* 'Col. Y.' (159) must be Colonel Lacy Yea, also killed at the Redan.

'H.V.' (153) would be Captain Hedley Vicars, who was killed bravely fighting back a Russian attack on his trench; his heroism and zealous faith were celebrated by Catherine Marsh in *Memorials of Captain Hedley Vicars*.

---

[12] George Eyre-Todd, ed., *The Autobiography of William Simpson* 57.

Dr John Hall, inspector general of hospitals, is the exception; Seacole identifies him by name and title while referencing a letter said to be written by him, a contentious claim that will be examined in Chapter 5.

In *Wonderful Adventures*, Seacole described looking after one — only one — patient in bed:

> one poor boy in the Artillery, with blue eyes and light golden hair, whom I nursed through a long and weary sickness, borne with all a man's spirit, and whom I grew to love like a fond old-fashioned mother (153).

She gave no specifics as to his illness or what she did for him. She took him into her own quarters, for she had no beds for patients or anybody else, for that matter. She mused that 'if ever angels watched over any life, they would shelter his,' but 'after he had left his sick bed, he was struck down on his battery.' She saw him buried (153).

Seacole claimed some success against bowel diseases, citing testimonial letters. She 'cured' a patient of 'very bad diarrhea' 'before the next morning' with her 'good medicine,' while another patient 'became quite well' in two days (128). Another who was 'severely attacked by diarrhea' was 'cured effectually' with but one dose of her medicine (129), and yet another she 'restored to health' (130). Her 'bitter sherry' made a successful remedy (130).

She claimed to have 'completely cured' in a month a 'severe inflammation of the chest,' which had persisted for four months, using (unspecified) 'medicine.' She 'restored to health' a patient with jaundice and claimed another cure for a 'severe attack of cholera in a few hours,' method not mentioned (131). Cholera was a 'visitor' to camp again late in the war, but, while she 'prescribed for many,' she claimed no successes at the time (150). 'We had cholera raging around us, carrying off its victims of all ranks' (160). A patient later expressed 'gratitude' to her for the 'kindness' received when ill (194).

In addition to Seacole's own account of her Crimean experiences, there are occasional references to her in the many war memoirs, journals and notes published by doctors, officers and visitors to the war. The artist William Simpson, who sketched her, observed in his autobiography:

> Mrs Seacole, an elderly mulatto woman from Jamaica, was a well-known character in the Crimea — all the soldiers and sailors knew her. She had a

taste for nursing and doctoring, but she added to this a business as a sutler. She told me one day that she had Scotch blood in her veins. I must say that she did not look like it, but the old lady spoke proudly of this point in her genealogy. She was a nice, good, creature, and everyone liked her.[13]

Lady Alicia Blackwood, wife of an army chaplain, reported favourably on the 'far-famed Mrs Seacole,' whose establishment was near their 'vicarage,' by the railway:

> she had wisely pitched her tent equally close to it on the opposite side or the line being used for the transport of goods and material from the port to the front. Doubtless she had a view to facilitating the transport of her stores also to her warehouse. Mrs Seacole kept a perfect Omnibus Shop, which was greatly frequented.

Blackwood credited her further with 'tact and never-varying good nature' for 'all her customers.' Her prices were 'heavy,' but no one grumbled for, in the distress of battle, she

> personally spared no pains and no exertion to visit the field of woe and minister with her own hands such things as could comfort or alleviate the sufferings of those around her, freely giving to such as could not pay, and to many whose eyes were closing in death, from whom payment could never be expected.[14]

An officer of the 46th South Devonshire Foot Guards noted lunches at Mrs Seacole's in his diary. For a Christmas treat for his troops he bought plum pudding ingredients from her.[15] He described seeing her at a magnificent march of 35,000 troops before General Codrington, along with the French commander General Pélissier and French and Sardinian troops:

> The French were delighted with the review and the Sardinians were in ecstasies. Mrs Seacole was there with a cart full of grub, but none of us poor regimental officers could get near it (207).

---

[13] Eyre-Todd, ed., *The Autobiography of William Simpson* 57.

[14] Alicia Blackwood, *Narrative of Personal Experiences and Impressions during a Residence on the Bosphorus throughout the Crimean War* 263.

[15] Colin Robins, ed., *Captain Dunscombe's Diary: The Real Crimean War That the British Infantry Knew* 188.

That Seacole's establishment was strictly for officers is made clear in the memoir by Colonel Sir James Alexander. Officers supervising works were 'not to refresh themselves at Mrs Seacole's store,' but 'to keep the men in sight the whole time' lest they 'steal off to public houses in Kadekoi.'[16]

A navy chaplain, soon after the war, published comments on his happy association with Mrs Seacole in the *United Service Magazine* (the next extract). He described her partner as 'a mild, unassuming individual.' She, on the other hand, was 'a large, unwieldy-looking woman, whose bark is worse than her bite. Her voice is harsh, but her heart is soft, and she has a good deal of the milk of human kindness in her bosom.' He remarked on the 'wags of the camp' referring to the firm of Seacole and Day as 'Day and Martin,' a racial joke playing on the fact that Martin was the name of a well-known black shoe polish. Seacole also quoted the wags' comment in her memoir (81). He gave a short chapter to her 'iron house' near the Col, a 'foreign provision store.' He noted her Creole birth and said she was 'of a strong mind and anti-slavery principles.'

She 'held a levee every morning after breakfast,' when 'sick men of every nation belonging to the Land Transport Corps' came in 'for a preventive against cholera, fever or the other incidental illnesses of the place.' He also reported her telling him, in a mysterious manner, about a troubling visit by three Americans to the English camp.

From: Arthur William Alsager Pollock, 'Reminiscences of the War in the East by a Military Chaplain,' *United Service Magazine* 339 (January 1857):97

Three Americans had just paid a sort of official visit to the English camp, and it was her positive opinion that they intended to hand her over bodily to the Russians at the earliest opportunity. She wished for my advice under the circumstances, and I endeavoured to disperse her fears, but she did not feel easy in her mind until they had left. She always expressed to me the utmost contempt for that nation; this was,

[16] James Edward Alexander, *Life of a Soldier, or Military Service in the East and West* 2:233.

no doubt, on account of their notions on slavery, for, having some African blood in her veins, she remembered the wrongs of her people. Americans were also in the habit of addressing her as the 'yaller woman' and, though the old lady was yellow enough, she did not like to be reminded of it. It was very amusing to hear her talk of her various expeditions to the different camps.//

Pollock, however, was given to exaggeration. For example, he reported an Artillery officer as describing her as 'a grand purveyor to the army, doctor of medicine, cook, confectioner and nurse — in fact quite a Caleb Quotem [Jack of all trades] in her way.' Another exaggeration was his contention that she had travelled 'almost' round the world, including Australia and California, places she never mentioned having visited (97).

The battlefield

Seacole's first view of battle took place when she rode with Omar Pasha and some Turkish troops towards a Russian outpost. She enjoyed it 'amazingly.' The advance on the Russians was a 'very pretty sight,' and the experience gave her a 'strange excitement' and longing to see more of warfare (147–48).

For the next battles, Seacole was ready for business. Many were the surmises as to when the expected assault on the Redan would take place, which happened on 18 June 1855, the anniversary of the Battle of Waterloo in 1815, when Wellington decisively beat Napoleon I.

Seacole reported that 'whispers were afloat on the evening' before (155). Also the day before, Sir Evelyn Wood, with other officers, had stopped at Seacole's hut, where they bought 'some bottled fruit, which we laughingly agreed should be kept for the survivors of the assault.'[17] That

---

[17] Evelyn Wood, *The Crimea in 1854 and 1894* 294; he was wounded severely at Redan; the quotation is from a section titled 'Unsuccessful assaults.'

evening Seacole and her staff prepared supplies for a pre-dawn departure: 'We were all busily occupied in cutting bread and cheese and sandwiches, packing up fowls, tongues and ham, wine and spirits' (156).

These were packed upon two mules, 'in charge of my steadiest lad.' She took with her a 'large bag, which I always carried into the field...with lint, bandages, needles, thread and medicines.' She duly led the way on horseback to Cathcart's Hill, which was 'crowded with non-combatants' (156). Seacole herself took what provisions she could carry to reach the reserves of Sir Henry Barnard's division, but, when they found that the Redan attack had failed, 'very wisely abstained.' Officers wanted her refreshments, and some wounded men 'found the contents of my bag very useful' (157).

When she got back to Cathcart's Hill, she found her horse but 'heard that the good-for-nothing lad' had gone away with the mules. She rode three miles after him and used her horse whip on him (158).

Seacole's next observation of actual battle was that of the Tchernaya, when the Russian Army attacked French and Sardinian positions on 16 August 1855. She was 'prepared and loaded as usual' and rode off to see 'the chief part of the morning's battle' (164). She described much plundering of bodies when she was attending to the wounds 'of many French and Sardinians,' helping to lift them into ambulances. She described tending the wounds of 'several Russians,' one of whom bit her when he died (166). She also looted, picking up 'some trophies from the battlefield, but not many, and those of little value.' She did not like 'plundering either the living or the dead, but I picked up a Russian metal cross.' She cut souvenir buttons off the coats of dead Russians (167).

A French soldier sold her a picture of a Madonna cut from the altar of a church in Sebastopol, eight or ten feet in length, which she took back with her to England (176). She paid another French soldier to bring the colt of a dead Cossack to her hut, made a pet of it and took it back also with her (167).

The army bombarded Sebastopol for some days in September in preparation for the final assault. 'Scarce a night passed that I was not lulled to sleep with the heavy continuous roar of the artillery,' she recalled (168). Rumours flew about a possible last effort the Russians would make 'to drive us into the sea.' She spent much of her time on

Cathcart's Hill watching. She also took a day off to attend a ceremony for the awarding of the Order of the Bath to senior officers, for which she sent a cake to headquarters, which was much appreciated (168–69).

One night during the bombardment, Seacole could not sleep and went out to watch:

> I thought the end of the world, instead of the war, was at hand when every battery opened and poured a perfect hail of shot and shell upon the beautiful city which I had left the night before sleeping so calm and peaceful beneath the stars.

The firing from early dawn made sleep impossible, so Seacole went to watch at Cathcart's Hill, where she provided refreshments to the spectators, 'right glad of any excuse to witness the last scene of the siege' (169). She noted, presumably a few days later, a change in weather, so that it was cold and wintry for 'the memorable 8th of September.' The Russians, apparently, had expected that the final assault would be made on 7 September, the anniversary of the Battle of Borodino of 1812, when the French lost one-third of their forces, the beginning of the end of Napoleon's 'Grande Armée.'[18] She went out with bandages and refreshments to her old spot. The cannonade stopped at noon, when the French come out of their trenches to move up to the Malakhoff. As in the first Redan attack in June, they held it briefly. The British attack on the Redan, as before, failed. The noon starting point of the infantry assault was to take advantage of the Russian change of shift.

Seacole was soon too busy to see much, for the wounded were more numerous than in the previous Redan assault. Slightly hurt stragglers 'limped in' and engrossed their attention. 'I now and then found time to ask them rapid questions, but they did not appear to know anything more than that everything had gone wrong' (170). She saw many of her officer friends of the 97th wounded and she dressed the wounds of several (170–71). The Russians continued to shell the allies and Seacole recounted being frightened, but 'afterwards I picked up a piece of this huge shell and brought it home

---

[18] Figes, *Crimea: The Last Crusade* 387.

with me' (171). Also on the battlefield, after the assault, she saw *The Times* correspondent, W.H. Russell, 'eagerly taking down notes and sketches of the scene.' He noticed her and mentioned her in his dispatch. He included the vignette also in his letter to the editor promoting the Seacole Fund after the war,[19] which she transcribed into her *Wonderful Adventures* (171–72).

The fall of Sebastopol

Much is made of Seacole having been the first British woman to enter Sebastopol on its fall, but the French vivandières were also quick to arrive and set up shop and may have been earlier. A British Army doctor walking through the city, who did not apparently encounter Seacole, reported seeing several French vivandières selling their wares.[20] The ending of the war was actually quite tame. There was no final battle, for the Russians, after enduring days of devastating bombardment by the allies, the destruction of most of the city and increasing desertions, simply walked out in the night of 8–9 September. They took many of their sick and wounded, but left hundreds of dead and dying soldiers, both in hospital and some in an unmarked departure shed. They scuttled their ships and set much of the city on fire. Seacole would have seen an abandoned and largely destroyed city, but there were no casualties in taking it. (Nightingale's cousin, Lothian Nicholson, a Royal Engineer, took part in the destruction of the port.)

Seacole's role at Sebastopol was her usual one of supplying food and drink. She obtained a signed note 'to pass Mrs Seacole and attendants with refreshments for officers and soldiers in Redan and Sebastopol,' signed by Major-General Robert Garrett (173). She had to borrow mules, for hers were exhausted from supplying spectators the previous night. She loaded them 'with good things' and set out 'with my partner and some

---

[19] From our special correspondent, 'The Fall of Sebastopol,' *The Times* 26 September 1855 8A; W.H.R., 'The Seacole Fund,' *The Times* 11 May 1857 8D.

[20] Frederick Robinson, *Diary of the Crimean War* 397.

other friends early on that memorable Sunday morning' [9 September 1855]. The travelling party stopped to give refreshments 'to officers and men' who had been without food for hours (173–74).

She took few of the 'many trophies' offered her by plundering soldiers. One, a 'decorated altar candle, studded with gold and silver stars,' she gave to the duke of Cambridge (174). The city was still burning in places.

Seacole described going into the city again on the following day, when she saw 'still more of its horrors,' but she 'refrained from describing so many scenes of woe,' 'where thousands of dead and dying had been left by the retreating Russians.' She wished that she had 'never seen that harrowing sight.' She understood that 'some Englishmen were found in it alive, but it was as well that they did not live to tell their fearful experience' (176–77).

Note that, while Seacole reported looking in at the hospital, she did not say anything about treating the sick or comforting the dying. Accounts by doctors and officers mention thousands left behind, the stench appalling.[21] Soyer called it 'one of the most awful and sickening sights possible for humanity to conjure up' and described 'hundreds of Russians, dead and dying,' uncared for, in dreadful agony, 'piled up one on the other, or lying singly on the bare flooring' (384).

After the taking of Sebastopol, there were no further battles, but peace negotiations proceeded slowly. The Russians still controlled the north side of the harbour and were by no means beaten. The French became increasingly desperate for peace as their death rates (from disease) rose in the second year of the war. The British Army was now well clothed and sheltered, and its food was immensely improved. Nightingale worked on getting more (non-drinking) leisure pursuits arranged for the men, such as reading and coffee rooms, one named the 'Inkermann Cafe.' Seacole herself referred to the coffee rooms (162).

An accidental explosion at a French Artillery Park on 13 November 1855 wounded and killed many. Seacole was observed by an officer 'hastening' to the scene in her cart:

---

[21] See, for example, George Ranken. *Six Months at Sebastopol* 72.

This was Mrs Seacole, who lived near the railway below Kadikoi and kept a sort of general store. She was a wonderful woman, a native of the West Indies, and had travelled over half the world. All the men swore by her, and in case of any malady would seek her advice and use her herbal medicines in preference to reporting themselves to their own doctors. That she did effect some cures is beyond doubt and her never failing presence among the wounded after a battle and assisting them made her beloved by the rank and file of the whole army. What became of her after we all sailed from the Crimea I never heard, but she carried away many a blessing with her wherever she may have gone.[22]

Officers had time for excursions, sports and dining, and Seacole obliged. 'Pleasure was hunted keenly,' she reported, to be found in 'cricket matches, picnics, dinner parties, races, theatricals....My restaurant was always full' (178). She provided soup and fish, turkeys, saddle of mutton, fowls, ham, tongue, curry, pastry of many sorts, custards, jelly, blancmange and olives (179), also 'cold duck...some cold meats, a tart' (190). There were accidents at the races, which meant patients for Seacole (182). A newspaper story of a race which described her as having 'presided over a sorely invested tentfull of creature comforts' noted that she was the 'only representative of the fair sex' attending.[23]

A Guards officer recounted a cricket match played against the 'Leg of Mutton Club,' which consisted of 'a medley of all sorts of regiments.'

We had a capital lunch on the ground, provided by an old black woman who kept a sort of eating house on the heights, and rejoiced in the appropriate and endearing title of 'Mother Sea Coal,' a native of Jamaica, and frightful to a degree, but a very clever 'doctress' on dit [it is said].[24]

In a late visit Soyer made to Seacole, he called her the 'mère noire,' a play on the French words for black mother and Black Sea, 'Mer Noire.' The second of the two excerpts immediately following relates a meeting he had with Nightingale at the hospital soon afterwards, when he passed on Seacole's 'kind inquiries.'

---

[22] F.H.D. Vieth, *Recollections of the Crimean Campaign* 74–75.

[23] 'The British Expedition,' *The Times* 17 December 1855 7A.

[24] Astley, *Fifty Years of my Life* 145.

From: Alexis Soyer, *Culinary Campaign* 434–35 and 436

I made it my duty to pay my respects to the illustrious Mrs Seacole and, like a good son or a ship in full sail, I was immediately received in the arms of the mère noire.... 'Hallo, my son! I saw you at headquarters yesterday!...Don't forget, before you go, to come and take a parting glass with an old friend. Mr Day and myself will be very glad to see you, depend upon it. By the way, how is Miss Nightingale?'

'I thank you, she was quite well the last time I had the pleasure of seeing her. I have to meet her at the Land Transport Hospital this morning, by appointment.'

'What nice kitchens those are of yours at the Land Transport Hospital! I saw them several times, and the doctors and Mrs Stuart [Jane Shaw Stewart] are highly pleased with them....You must know, M Soyer, that Miss Nightingale is very fond of me. When I passed through Scutari, she very kindly gave me board and lodging.' This was about the twentieth time the old lady had told me the same tale.

She [Nightingale] said, with a smile, 'I should like to see her [Seacole] before she leaves, as I hear she has done a deal of good for the poor soldiers.' 'She has indeed, I assure you, and with the greatest disinterestedness. While I was there this morning, she was dressing a poor Land Transport Corps man who had received a severe contusion on the head. In order to strengthen his courage for the process, as she said, she made him half a glass of strong brandy and water, not charging him anything for it, and I hear she has done this repeatedly.' 'I am sure she has done much good.'//

Soyer also told Lord William Paulet, the commandant, that Seacole was 'an excellent woman, kind to everybody, I can assure you' (299). He agreed.

Seacole's last accounts of her war excursions and partings are touching. She was given presents and many expressions of thanks (193). Press coverage shows that she was well enough known to be mentioned for the most mundane events. One story reported that 'Mrs Seacole, who keeps a restaurant near the Col, avers that a piece of stone struck her door, which is three and a half or four miles from the park.'[25] A later story reported her having made 'the grand tour by Bakshiserai and Simpheropol,' noting that she had 'managed to leave some of her stock behind her.' It goes on that 'the sultan has sent her a medal, but she is anxiously expecting the English government to decorate her with the Crimean riband and its metallic appendage'[26] (the metallic appendage refers to the clasps awarded for specific battles and the siege). However, her memoir records no receipt of any medal. An item a few weeks later reported that troops marching past gave Seacole a cheer.[27]

Troops, with their officers, were moved back to England as soon as possible after the signing of the peace treaty. Seacole and Day, however, could not sell their (expanded) stock at a decent price. Expensive cheeses went for a tenth their cost. Seacole took a hammer to cases of red wine to keep the Russians from getting them for free (196). No one would pay money for the huts, which were torn down. The firm of Seacole and Day had to declare bankruptcy, which was duly granted the following year back in England.

Shortly before leaving the Crimea, Soyer took a last glimpse 'at the ruins of the Seacole Tavern' (479). If this is irreverent, his final words on her, soon after, were not: she was 'among the group of lookers-on...the illustrious Mrs Seacole, dressed in a riding habit, and for the last time this excellent mother was bidding farewell to all her sons, thus ending her benevolent exertions in the Crimea' (482).

Did Seacole have a fourteen-year-old daughter with her in the Crimea? Her memoir makes no mention of one, but her friend Soyer unambiguously called the girl staying with her 'Miss Sally Seacole' (269), or 'her daughter, Sarah,' whom he reverted back to calling 'Sally' (435). The girl is not mentioned in any later references to Seacole, nor in

---

[25] 'The British Expedition,' *The Times* 4 December 1855 7D.

[26] 'The British Army,' *The Times* 16 May 1856 10C.

[27] 'The British Army,' *The Times* 9 June 1856 10B.

her will. Seacole twice mentioned having a 'little girl' with her in Panama, but gave no name for her, nor their relationship (*WA* 12 and 36). One biographer thought that Thomas Day was likely Sarah Seacole's father.[28] The two census records available for Seacole, 1871 and 1881, show no Sarah Seacole living with her.

Seacole's departure date from the Crimea is unknown. She took a circuitous route on a 'crowded steamer' (197) and was back in England early in July 1856.

Post-Crimea, back in England

Seacole continued to get good press coverage on her return to England. Even the stories about the bankruptcy treat her with respect. She was always 'Mrs Seacole,' a 'lady,' and compliments abound. She knew how to play the press, who seem to have been happy to oblige. The source used here is *The Times*, which, as a conservative, imperialist paper, would be close to Seacole's own views.

Early in July 1856 there was a story about her plan to open a store at Aldershot, where the British Army had a major base:

> Mrs Seacole, the celebrated proprietress of the provision store in the Crimea, intends setting up a similar establishment at Aldershot. Her fame in that particular department of business is so well known among all military men that success in her new speculation is almost certain.[29]

A *Punch* item the next day noted her plan to set up 'a store at Aldershot, where I have little doubt she will attract crowds' (6 July 1856, 3).

In August, Seacole was an 'illustrious' visitor to a dinner at Surrey Gardens. Her appearance 'awakened the most rapturous enthusiasm. The soldiers not only cheered her, but chaired her around the gardens.'[30] In

---

[28] Ron Ramdin, *Mary Seacole* 123.

[29] 'Mrs Seacole,' *The Times* 5 July 1856 10C.

[30] 'The Dinner to the Guards,' *The Times* 26 August 1856 7C.

September, her presence was noted at a similar dinner in Portsmouth, for which Nightingale's father was said to have given a handsome donation and a hamper of game.[31]

She presumably did not attend the annual Woolwich Garrison Races in October, or her presence would likely have been noted. This event included foot races for non-commissioned officers and men, who ran a distance of 300 yards, without boots, stripped to their shirts and drawers. For the officers there were horse races. The third race was won by a brown filly, 'Mrs Seacole,' for the Benefit Stakes of five sovereigns each, with £40 added.[32] Another story added that 'Mrs Seacole made steady running throughout and won, after a good race, by half a length.'[33]

Bankruptcy proceedings regarding Seacole and Day, provision merchants, began in November 1856. The first item is revealing as it gives the earliest description of her wearing army medals — they do not appear in *Wonderful Adventures*:

> Mrs Seacole is a lady of colour and has been honoured with four government medals for her kindness to the British soldiery. She was present in person and attracted much attention, the gaily coloured decorations on her breast being in perfect harmony with the rest of her attire.[34]

The first of several sympathetic letters to the editor about her situation was by an anonymous Da Meritis.[35] The second, a reply to it, was by her great supporter, Lord Rokeby, announcing a subscription to aid her to 'recommence the business to which she is accustomed.'[36]

---

[31] 'The Portsmouth Crimean Banquets,' *The Times* 15 September 1856 12B.

[32] 'Woolwich Garrison Races,' *The Times* 22 October 1856 10A.

[33] *Racing Times* 27 October 1856 343.

[34] 'Bankruptcy Court: In re Seacole and Day,' *The Times* 7 November 1856 9B.

[35] 'Mrs Seacole A Bankrupt,' *The Times* 24 November 1856 8F.

[36] *The Times* 25 November 1856 6F.

Another supporter suggested that the newspaper publish her address so that people could forward money to her.[37] The next day another supporter, who had known her in the Crimea and since seen her in London, wrote urging that people send their contributions for 'this good old lady...for the purpose of re-establishing her in business, as soon as her certificate from the Court of Bankruptcy is granted.'[38] Lord Rokeby wrote again, this time including a letter from Seacole herself,[39] which will be reprinted shortly.

A women's paper published a highly sympathetic story about her bankruptcy: 'Mrs Seacole's bankruptcy has elicited many expressions of regret from those who were witnesses of her exertions and acts of benevolence as vivandière of the British Army in the Crimea.' It added that a *Times* correspondent writing from the Reform Club gave £20 to start contributions from 'the Crimeans.'[40]

Bankruptcy court hearings in 1857 got brief mentions in the press.[41] Her business partner, Thomas Day, wrote a letter to the editor about the causes of the bankruptcy, clarifying specifically that officers owing money, as Russell had alleged in his letter, was not a significant factor, but rather the bankruptcy could be attributed to 'losses by the elements,' robbery and depreciation of their 'stock in trade and buildings.'[42] There were newspaper advertisements for the sale of pictures of Seacole as 'Mother of the British Army.' [43]

---

[37] Letter from H. Fane Keane, *The Times* 27 November 1856 7E.

[38] *The Times* 28 November 1856 8A.

[39] 'Mrs Seacole,' *The Times* 29 November 1856 12D.

[40] *The Lady's Newspaper* London 29 November 1856 349.

[41] *The Times* 8 January 1857 11E, 9 January 1857 9B, 31 January 1857 11B, and 28 August 1857 9C.

[42] 'Mrs Seacole's Late Partner in the Crimea,' *The Times* 14 April 1857 7F.

[43] 'Mrs Seacole,' *The Times* 2 July 1857 1A.

The first Seacole Fund, 1857

A number of leading officers came to Seacole's rescue when her financial difficulties became known. A fundraising committee was formed and fundraising in earnest began as soon as the bankruptcy certificate was granted. The following list gives the names of committee members, with a note of any financial contribution they are known to have made and, for two, their membership also on the later committee.

1857 Seacole committee[44]
Maj Gen Lord Rokeby, chair, treasurer, gave £10, also on 1867 committee
Prince Edward of Saxe Weimar, gave £1 in 1867
Duke of Newcastle, gave £10
Duke of Wellington, gave £10
Lord Ward, gave £25
Gen Sir J.F. Burgoyne
Maj Gen Sir Richard Airey, quartermaster general
Rear Adm Sir Stephen Lushington, gave £2.2.0 in 1867
Col McMurdo, director general, Military Train
Col Chapman, R.E.
Lt Col Ridley
Maj the Hon F. Keane, also on 1867 committee, and gave £2
W.H. Russell, late special correspondent, *The Times*
W.T. Doyne, late superintendent general, Army Works Corps
Honorary secretaries: Chapman and Doyne.

The Surrey Gardens festivities put on in Seacole's honour in July 1857 were well attended and well covered in the press. The first of many stories on the concerts explained that the money was 'to put her beyond the reach

---

[44] 'The Seacole Fund,' *The Times* 13 June 1857 9A; 30 January 1867 5B; 11 March 1867 5B.

of want.'[45] A story the next day recounted 'the grand military festival for the benefit of Mrs Seacole,' where she 'sat in state.' The praise was lavish:

> At the end of both the first and the second parts, the name of Mrs Seacole was shouted by a thousand voices. The genial old lady rose from her place and smiled benignantly on the assembled multitude, amid a tremendous and continued cheering. Never did woman seem happier, and never was hearty and kindly greeting bestowed upon a worthier subject.[46]

The Times account on the last day of the festival was nearly as warm:

> At the end of the first part of the concert, there was a universal call for Mrs Seacole, who, to the surprise and satisfaction of everyone, was led forward in the orchestra by M Jullien [the conductor] with a gallantry as hearty as it was expressive. After the second part, in answer to a similarly enthusiastic summons, Mrs Seacole bowed her acknowledgments from her accustomed seat in the front gallery. This evening, the last of the festival, it is, we are informed, the intention of Mrs Seacole to address the audience.

Whether or not she did is not known. The story has a further point, that Seacole discussed going to India during the mutiny with Lord Panmure, the secretary for war.[47] However, there is no reference to any such meeting in *The Panmure Papers*, which reports much correspondence from the beginning of the mutiny but nothing on sending nurses. Nightingale had only recently sent Panmure her detailed proposal for women nurses in army hospitals, dated 3 May 1857.[48] A Seacole letter to Sir Henry Storks, military secretary at the War Office, emerged recently that requests him to peruse an enclosed letter (not now available) and 'kindly alter any part that might not meet your approval before

---

[45] 'The Seacole Festival at Royal Surrey Gardens,' *The Times* 27 July 1857 8F.

[46] 'Festival at the Royal Surrey Gardens,' *The Times* 28 July 1857 10D.

[47] 'The Seacole Festival,' *The Times* 30 July 1857 5F.

[48] George Douglas and George Dalhousie Ramsay, eds, *The Panmure Papers* 2:381–84.

returning it.[49,] However, not only is the draft letter to Panmure missing, there is nothing to suggest that Seacole ever sent any letter to him.

The possibility of Seacole going to the mutiny was turned into a performance, 'Another Volunteer for India,' with an actress playing Seacole as 'vivandière,' to the tune of 'Cheer, Boys, Cheer.'[50] In fact Seacole did not go, and there is no evidence that she ever tried to. Her sister told Anthony Trollope, when in Jamaica on government business, that Queen Victoria had stopped her because her life was 'too precious.' His account, from his stay at Blundell Hall in 1858, explains with rare detail the lodging house:

> I took up my abode at Blundle [Blundell] Hall, and found that the landlady in whose custody I had placed myself was a sister of good Mrs Seacole. 'My sister wanted to go to India,' said my landlady, 'with the army, you know. But Queen Victoria would not let her — her life was too precious.' So that Mrs Seacole is a prophet, even in her own country.[51]

He was not favourably impressed with West Indian hotels — the best hotel he experienced was in Cuba. He continued:

> This one, kept by Mrs Seacole's sister, was not worse, if not much better, than the average. It was clean and reasonable as to its charges. I used to wish that the patriotic lady who kept it could be induced to abandon the idea that beefsteaks and onions, and bread and cheese and beer, composed the only diet proper for an Englishman. But it is to be remarked, all through the island, that the people are fond of English dishes, and that they despise, or affect to despise, their own productions (21).

The humour magazine *Punch* published a letter Seacole wrote, in the third person, on her financial troubles. It was illustrated with a cartoon showing her taking copies of the magazine around to soldier patients, presumably at the Land Transport Hospital near her hut. The letter

---

[49] Elizabeth Anionwu, Corry Staring-Derks and Jeroen Staring, 'New Light on Seacole,' *Nursing Standard* 27,50 (14 August 2013):23.

[50] 'City of London Theatre,' *The Times* 28 December 1857 9D.

[51] Anthony Trollope, *The West Indies and the Spanish Main* 21.

humorously relates her woes. It also reveals her utter devotion to the imperial British cause, even the suggestion that she would go to China to serve — at the time of the disgraceful Opium Wars! No wonder the letter is not used in the Seacole campaign. Also noteworthy is the fact that Seacole never specified what she might do to help in China, except that it would be 'woman's work.' She makes no mention of nursing. The timing is also of interest, for the letter dates to May 1857, after the outbreak of the Indian Mutiny, to which, some Seacole supporters assert, Seacole wanted to go to nurse.

From: Seacole letter, 'Our Own Vivandière,' *Punch* 30 May 1857 221

Mother Seacole loves to acknowledge the kindness shown her by her sons, whether in black or red coats, and hastens to assure Punch that she has long felt a mother's affection for him. For she remembers a time when a word of cheer and encouragement from home broke like a ray of golden sunlight through the gloom of a suffering army, and that word Punch never failed to give her soldier sons. Nor has she forgotten how — as she walked through the wards of the hospital at Spring Hill — her arms laden with papers, the contributions of kind officers to their sick men, the sufferers would plead for a glimpse of Punch, which seldom failed to have a heart-stirring piece of poetry or a noble sketch in appreciation of their struggles. She has some of these numbers now, old and worn and frayed by many a strong hand brought low by the Russian bullet or pestilence. It shared the high popularity of the *Illustrated London News* and, remembering these old times, it stirs the heart of Mother Seacole like the sound of the old war cry she may never hear again, to find her poor name noticed in the columns which cheered on England to a noble contest.

And, more than this, Mother Seacole, in this her season of want — for the peace which brought blessings to so many ruined her — feels that the notice of her good son Punch brings sunshine into the poor little room — not quite a garret yet, thank God, she has one more weary storey to climb before her pallet rests so near the sky — to which she is reduced.

Not that the army's mother murmurs at her lot. She knows that she is not flung aside like — like some of the brave men for whose blood there is no further need — and she believes there will yet be work for her to do somewhere. Perhaps in China, perhaps on some other distant shore to which Englishmen go to serve their country, there may be woman's work to do — and for that work, if her good son Punch will cheer her on, old Mother Seacole has a heart and hands left yet.//

Nothing came of any of the possible campaigns mentioned; Seacole did not go to, or attempt to go to, China, or anywhere else where 'Englishmen go to serve their country.'

Seacole's memoir was probably published in late June or early July of 1857, as it began to be noted in the 'Books Received' sections of periodicals in early July, and a full review, possibly the first, appeared in mid-July.[52] A Dutch translation came out in 1857, *Mary Seacole's Avonturen in de West en in de Krim*, which was reprinted in 2007. A French translation appeared in 1858, *Aventures et voyages d'une Créole à Panama et en Crimée*, reprinted in 2011. The original book was an immediate success, sold out and was soon reprinted. The reaction to it and first reviews are related in Chapter 6.

Soyer saw Seacole one last time at a bazaar in London in January 1858, when he was near death. She was 'jolly Mother Seacole, stout and flourishing as ever.'[53]

A curious item in the *Teesdale Mercury* excerpts a note from a Brussels newspaper, the *Nord*, that 'Lady Seacole' arrived in Antwerp from London, adorned with 'all her decorations,' which it enumerated as the Legion of Honour, the English Crimean medal and the Medjidie. Seacole is further described as the 'companion of the

---

[52] *The Critic* 16,391 (15 July 1857):321–22.

[53] Morris, *Portrait of a Chef* 202.

celebrated Miss Nightingale.'[54] Neither the purpose nor the length of the visit are known. Given that Antwerp was then the closest port to Rotterdam, the location of her Dutch publishers, it is likely that she was going to meet with them.

Seacole continued to receive press attention. Visits she made in 1859 to the military bases at Sheerness had her receiving 'a hearty and kind welcome from the garrison officers,' as she did also at Chatham Barracks and Melville Hospital.[55]

Later in 1859, Seacole returned to Jamaica,[56] possibly on account of the inadequacy of the funds raised for her. Nothing is known of her activities for the next years there. She was spotted visiting Panama in 1863, as reported by an unnamed person who stopped there on a voyage. He described arriving at dusk and getting to his hotel, 'where we saw the sunny face of Mrs Seacole of Crimean renown, gadding about with naval officers on leave from the frigate *Orlando*.'[57]

Seacole returned to England in 1865.[58] Possibly she made further (undocumented) trips back and forth, but it seems that she settled in England in 1865 for good.

A cholera epidemic in England broke out in 1866 and was estimated to have caused some 6,000 deaths. Seacole contributed to a relief fund for it: '100 bottles of anti-cholera medicine and 100 boxes of pills,' contents not stated.[59] This is the only known contribution to health care in England Seacole is known to have made.

---

[54] 'Elevation of Mrs Seacole,' *Teesdale Mercury* 28 June 1858; a similar item appeared in the *Morning Advertiser* of 30 August 1858.

[55] 'Military and Naval Intelligence,' *The Times* 1 February 1859 10C.

[56] 'The Mails, &c, Southampton,' *The Times* 18 October 1859 6E.

[57] 'A Trip to Vancouver Island,' *United Service Magazine* No. 416 (July 1863):383.

[58] 'The West India and Pacific Mails,' *The Times* 14 October 1865 10G.

[59] 'Mansion House Cholera Relief Fund,' *The Times* 31 August 1866 6A.

The second Seacole Fund, 1867

The 1857 events at Surrey Gardens drew large crowds, but in the end, after expenses were paid, the profits were meagre. One story even suggested — an exaggeration — that Seacole received nothing from the proceeds.[60] A letter to the editor by the director of the Surrey Gardens corrected this, stating that she would receive the full amount owed,[61] which of course was not enough to support her. Another, lengthier explanation of what went wrong included quotations from the conductor of the music.[62]

A second committee, largely with new members, was formed in 1867 and was thoroughly successful. This time the names of three royal patrons preceded those of the ordinary committee members: the prince of Wales and the duke of Edinburgh, sons of Queen Victoria, and the duke of Cambridge, commander-in-chief of the army and a cousin of the queen.

On the committee were members of the nobility, other titled men, military officers (navy as well as army) and a few civilians. There were brigade and regimental commanders and adjutant generals; also Lord Frederick Paulet, brother of the commandant, Lord William Paulet. The big difference in 1867 was that Queen Victoria now gave her approbation and herself contributed (amount unspecified). The intermediary was Count Gleichen,[63] as Prince Victor of Hohenlohe-Langenburg a relative. A member of the Seacole Fund, he had been a customer at her store, as is related shortly.

---

[60] 'In Re the Surrey Gardens Company (Limited),' *The Times* 24 August 1857 9B.

[61] 'The Royal Surrey Gardens,' *The Times* 31 August 1857 6F.

[62] 'Royal Surrey Gardens Company,' *The Lady's Newspaper* 29 August 1857 134.

[63] Gleichen letters 23 and 25 January 1867; Thomas Biddulph letter to Gleichen 27 January 1867, Royal Archives, Windsor Castle PPTO/PP/QV/MAIN/1867/23078.

1867 Seacole committee[64]
Prince of Wales, patron
Duke of Edinburgh, patron
Duke of Cambridge, patron, gave £10 in 1857, £15 in 1867
Col Henry Daniell, chair of 1867 committee, £2.10.0 (Mrs Daniel £2.10.0)
Prince of Leiningen, gave £2.2.0
Count Gleichen, gave £2
Lord Frederick Paulet, gave £2
Viscount Dangan, gave £2
Adm the Hon Sir Henry Keppel, gave £3.3.0
Col G. Gambier, Royal Artillery
Capt F. Hawkins, gave £2
Col de Bathe, gave £2
Col G.W. Higginson, gave £2
Capt Walrond Clarke, gave £2
Lt Col W. McCall, honorary secretary of committee, gave £2
Plus Rokeby and Keane of the 1857 committee.

The fund also reported names of contributors and amounts, an impressive list. Distinguished givers included wealthy philanthropist Angela Burdett Coutts (£10) and Maj Gen the Hon [Robert] J. Lindsay, MP and VC (£2). There were several other MPs, VCs and MP VCs. There were anonymous donations, some sizable. The only doctor listed was Dr Young, HMS *Galatea*, who gave five shillings to the 1867 fund. A Dutch researcher has uncovered evidence of fundraising done for her in 1857 in Bristol, and in New Zealand in 1867.[65]

The original 1857 committee was clear that its purpose was not only to 'provide a fund sufficient to secure to this worthy woman a provision for the autumn of her life,' but to make it possible for 'her unimpaired habits of activity and industry' to be 'turned to good and useful

---

[64] 'The Seacole Fund,' *The Times* 30 January 1867 5B, 2 March 1867 8C, and 11 March 1867 5B.

[65] Jeroen Staring blog, posted 18 May 2013.

account.'[66] The same point about gainful employment was made in 1867, now less realistically, to 'ensure for Mrs Seacole, in her declining years, the means of obtaining remunerative employment, whereby competence would to her be secured.'[67] Russell's own words, in his preface to *Wonderful Adventures*, similarly implied future employment.

One fundraising event was held in 1867, the performance of a romantic drama, The Marble Heart, with a band concert.[68] Otherwise the fund was based on subscriptions.

Nightingale biographer Mark Bostridge uncovered evidence that Nightingale had contributed to the 1857 Seacole Fund, in a letter by an aunt to Nightingale's mother. In that letter, her aunt noted having seen Nightingale's name on a list of subscribers, although no such list is now to be found.[69] Published lists of contributors to the later fund include several from 'anonymous' and 'a lady,' so that the absence of a name on a list is not conclusive.

Seacole's appearances at public events continued to receive coverage in *The Times,* for example, when she was noticed sitting behind the witness box at a trial.[70] The sale of a portrait of her that year was advertised.[71]

Seacole's supporters

Three of Seacole's supporters were particularly important: W.H. Russell, Count Gleichen and Lord Rokeby; the latter two remained staunch

---

[66] 'The Seacole Fund,' *The Times* 13 June 1857 9A.

[67] 'The Seacole Fund,' *The Times* 30 January 1867 5B.

[68] 'The Wandering Thespians,' *The Times* 18 July 1867 8C.

[69] Mark Bostridge, *Florence Nightingale: The Woman and her Legend* 274; letter 6 August [1857], Claydon House bundle 309.

[70] 'The Jamaica Prosecutions,' *The Times* 13 February 1867 12C.

[71] 'Sales by Auction,' *The Times* 29 March 1867 16A.

supporters and became trustees for her will. Soyer of course was important during the war, but he had nothing to do with the Seacole Fund post-war and he died in 1858.

William Howard Russell (1821–1907)

Known as the 'first war correspondent,' W.H. Russell was a friend and supporter of Seacole. He had been a customer of hers and is listed among those with unpaid debts at the end of the war, albeit for an insignificant sum,[72] presumably repaid. He had a long and distinguished career as a war correspondent, covering notably the American Civil War. He was knighted in 1895.

Russell's commendation of Seacole became the central message of the fundraising campaign for her. He admired and respected her, but he did not make her quite the heroine today's campaigners suggest. His report on Seacole after the fall of Sebastopol was generous, saying that she 'doctors and cures all manner of men with extraordinary success' at her 'abode, an iron storehouse with wooden sheds and outlying tributaries.' He gave her credit for being 'in attendance near the battlefield,' and for earning 'many a poor fellow's blessing.'[73]

His preface to her memoir is even more generous, probably because of her need for funds — it was written just after bankruptcy proceedings began. It is often quoted, or rather partially quoted. A page long, the core of it states:

> If singleness of heart, true charity and Christian works, if trials and sufferings, dangers and perils, encountered boldly by a helpless woman on her errand of mercy in the camp and in the battlefield can excite sympathy or move curiosity, Mary Seacole will have many friends and many readers....

---

[72] 'Bankruptcy Court,' *The Times* 8 January 1857 11E.

[73] W.H. Russell, *The War: From the Death of Lord Raglan to the Evacuation of the Crimea* 187–88.

I have witnessed her devotion and her courage; I have already borne testimony to her services to all who needed them. She is the first who has redeemed the name of 'sutler' from the suspicion of worthlessness, mercenary baseness and plunder, and I trust that England will not forget one who nursed her sick, who sought out her wounded to aid and succour them, and who performed the last offices for some of her illustrious dead (vii-viii).

Seacole campaign supporters of today, however, typically omit mention of her main occupation of sutler, to cite only her (occasional) first aid work for soldiers.

Russell also wrote an appeal that appeared in April 1857 in *The Times*, explaining why she deserved a subscription. It ended:

I hope the public, as well as the army, will give enough to Mrs Seacole to set her up — late in life, poor soul! though it be, it is all she asks — for a fresh start in the world, and that, as she was liberal and kind, so may she receive a kind and liberal support.[74]

Of his hundreds of pages of dispatches from the war, only a few short sections go to Seacole. One story which mentioned her was reprinted in his second volume on the war.[75] His retrospective, *The Great War with Russia: The Invasion of the Crimea, 1895*, does not mention her, nor do compilations by later editors.[76] Seacole scarcely gets a mention in biographies on him.[77]

Russell was a member of the 1857 Seacole committee, but not of the 1867 committee, and one wonders if there was a reason for this, possibly the medals hoax. When he wrote his generous words about Seacole,

---

[74] W.H.R., 'The Seacole Fund,' *The Times* 11 April 1857 8D.

[75] *The War: From the Death of Lord Raglan to the Evacuation of the Crimea* 2:187–88, from the story in *The Times* 26 September 1855. His first collection, *The War: From the Landing at Gallipoli to the Death of Lord Raglan*, has no mention of her.

[76] *Despatches from the Crimea*, 1906; *Russell's Despatches from the Crimea*, 1966; *The Noise of Drums and Trumpets*, 1971; *Russell of The Times*, 1984.

[77] There is no mention of her in J.B. Atkins, *The Life of Sir William Howard Russell* or Rupert Furneaux, *The First War Correspondent: William Howard Russell*; there is a brief note only in Alan Hankinson, *Man of Wars: William Howard Russell* 103.

perhaps she had not begun to wear the medals, or he did not know that she did. Possibly he was offended by her doing so.

Count Gleichen, Prince Victor Hohenlohe-Langenburg (1833–91)

Count Gleichen, as he was known to Seacole, was the son of Queen Victoria's half-sister, a captain in the Royal Navy and an amateur sculptor. He appears in her memoir as a customer at her store, 'one of my kindest customers, a lieutenant serving in the Royal Naval Brigade, who was a close relative of the queen, whose uniform he wore.' He called her 'Mami' for their acquaintance had begun in Jamaica. Gleichen approached Seacole over a problem of fly infestation — he told her they 'make a supper of me.' There was not much she could do, but she procured a piece of muslin which she pinned up into a mosquito net for him and 'the prince was delighted.' He fell ill later that summer and Seacole 'went up to his quarters and did all I could for him' (163–64).

Gleichen was a member of the 1867 Seacole Fund, but his greatest contribution was the terracotta sculpture he made of her in 1871, 'adorned with her Crimean medals.'[78] The bust, apparently shown at the Royal Academy of Arts summer exhibition the following year, is now at the Institute of Jamaica. A copy of the bust was made by George Kelly.

As a naval officer and relative of Queen Victoria, Gleichen must have known that the three large medals and the brooch of the Order of the Medjidie, prominent on the bust, were not Seacole's. Challen probably knew too that the three medals he painted on her were not hers, but Gleichen was a military man so that his sculpture of her proudly wearing four is more than puzzling.

Seacole left Gleichen the same £50 bequest she gave her other trustees, plus 'Nelson's diamond ring.' She left his eldest daughter her 'best set of pearl ornaments,' and nineteen guineas each to the other children.

---

[78] 'Sculpture in the Studio,' *The Times* 21 July 1871 4E.

Lieutenant General Lord Rokeby (1798–1883)

Born Henry Robinson Montagu, the 6th Baron Rokeby, KCB, started the first Seacole Fund and remained Seacole's supporter until her death. She dedicated *Wonderful Adventures* to him. He explained, in a letter to *The Times*, that she had called on him in mid-November 1856, requesting advice and assistance. He undertook to promote a subscription 'to enable her to recommence the business to which she is accustomed,' after she obtained a certificate from the Court of Bankruptcy. He had the name of Sir Henry Barnard and had retained Messrs Cox to receive the money.[79] She thanked him in a letter which he sent to the editor of *The Times*, with another by him, both of which it published; Seacole's is reproduced here.

From: 'Mrs Seacole,' *The Times* 29 November 1856 12D

No. 1 Tavistock Street

25 November [1856]

My Lord, With much gratitude I beg to offer you my sincere thanks for your letter, which I have just read in *The Times* of today, and would publicly acknowledge your present as well as past kindnesses to me, but I fancy you, my Lord, might object to my placing your name in the public papers; consequently I take this means of expressing to you my gratitude for the interest you take in my case.

I am fully aware of the kind feelings yourself and the army have towards me, and this knowledge tends to sustain me in my present difficulties, and, far from regretting my visit to the Crimea, I feel proud indeed that I have had an opportunity to gain the esteem of your Lordship, along with that of many others in the army, and indeed I would much rather suffer my present poverty with the knowledge

---

[79] 'To the Editor of *The Times*,' *The Times* 25 November 1856 6F.

that the Almighty permitted me to be useful in my small sphere, than have returned wealthy without the esteem and regard of the brave defenders of our country.

Trusting your Lordship will excuse the liberty I have taken in thus writing to your Lordship, I am your Lordship's

very humble and grateful servant

Mary Seacole

To the Right Hon Lord Rokeby, M[ajor] G[eneral]

Portman Square, London//

Lord Rokeby was still a trustee of the Seacole Fund at her death when he received a bequest of £50 'as a slight mark of my gratitude for his many kindnesses to me, to purchase a ring if he so pleases.'

Two other supporters of lesser importance to the above three were:

Lord George Paget (1818–80), after Lord Cardigan, commander of the Light Brigade in the Crimean War. He notably sat beside Seacole, with Rokeby on the other side, at one of the Surrey Gardens events.[80] His letters and journal, however, make no reference to her, nor to Nightingale, although he did praise the 'admirable manner' that Jane Shaw Stewart, the superintendent of nursing at the Castle Hospital, conducted the nursing there.[81]

Captain the Hon H. Fane Keane (1822–95), a Royal Engineer, later General, CB, was a member of both fundraising committees. He, as a trustee of Seacole's will, was left £50 'for some ornament or jewel.' He was described by *The Times* war correspondent as chiefly passing his time 'preparing cooling drinks at Mrs Seacole's.'[82]

---

[80] 'Festival at the Royal Surrey Gardens,' *The Times* 28 July 1857 10D.

[81] Paget, *The Light Cavalry Brigade of the Crimea* 106.

[82] Russell letter, Hankinson, *Man of Wars* 103.

Retirement years, conversion and death

Seacole, on her return from Jamaica in 1865, spent her retirement years in England, in comfort at least from 1867, thanks to the funds raised for her. It seems that she did not work again after the Crimean War, apart from the very brief attempt at running a shop at Aldershot. There is anecdotal evidence that she was, on her return, masseuse to the princess of Wales, later Queen Alexandra, but the documentation is weak (the queen's own papers were destroyed). A letter to the editor of a Jamaican newspaper reported, in 1938, that she had made her living as a 'rubber,' or masseuse, to the princess, some thirty years after the war. That same account, however, had her wearing 'a dozen medals.'[83] Another letter to the editor reported that Seacole arranged to have mangoes on ice sent from Jamaica for the princess (Seacole was friendly with the superintendent of the Royal Mail Steamship Co.).[84] The mango shipment is dated to 1873, but the letter appeared only in 1939, sixty-six years after the event in question.

In the 1871 census, when Seacole was living at 40 Upper Berkeley St., St Marylebone, she reported her occupation as 'annuitant.'[85]

She evidently wore medals when she walked about London. Dr Douglas A. Reid reported seeing her wearing one, which he took to have been awarded her by 'the authorities, in recognition of her benevolent services':

> Some years afterwards I met her at Charing Cross. The medal first attracted my eye, and on looking up I recognised her dusky countenance. Of course I stopped her, and we had a short talk together about Crimean times. She had a store at Kadikoi, near Balaclava, for some time, where she sold all sorts of

---

[83] Major A.C. Whitehorne, letter *The Daily Gleaner* 5 February 1938.

[84] Mrs K. Stewart, 'Jamaica's Florence Nightingale,' *The Gleaner* 25 August 1939.

[85] *Census Returns of England and Wales*, 1871, National Archives; http://search.ancestry.ca/cgi-bin/sse.dll?h+289335188db=uk1871&indiv=try.

commodities, clothing and articles of food that were luxuries to us. I need not say that she was largely patronized.[86]

In the 1881 census, about a month before her death, Seacole was living at 3 Cambridge St., Paddington, occupation listed as 'independent.'[87]

The fact that she sought burial in a Roman Catholic cemetery suggests that Seacole converted at some point. She did not describe her faith, or any church attendance, in her memoir. Chaplains (Church of England and Roman Catholic) held services in the Crimea, but Seacole never mentioned attending any.

Only the most cursory and conventional references to 'God' and 'Providence' appear in her memoir. In Cruces, she prayed that God would spare the life of an orphan infant with cholera, 'but it did not please him to grant my prayer' (29). In relating her desire to go to the Crimea, Seacole quoted Jesus, 'I was sick and ye visited me' (75) from Matthew 25:35. Near the end of the Crimean War, she said that she did not 'pray God that I may never see its like again' (159). On the day the allies entered Sebastopol, a French soldier sold her a (looted) painting of the Madonna. With its 'look of divine calmness and heavenly love,' she imagined that, during the siege, 'many a knee was bent in worship before it, and many a heart found comfort in its soft loving gaze' (176). On a cemetery visit shortly before leaving the Crimea, she reflected on her friends, praying gratefully to 'Providence' for taking some and in mercy sparing the rest (195). Not a word about her conversion is available, nor any other information about her faith.

Seacole died of apoplexy on 14 May 1881 at her home in London, at age seventy-six, according to the death certificate. *The Times* obituary,

---

[86] Reid, *Memories of the Crimean War* 14. This memoir also devotes some space to recounting Nightingale's work.

[87] *Census Returns of England and Wales*, 1881, National Archives of the UK. RG10, 165,64,7. http://search.ancestry.ca/cgi-bin/sse.dll?h+289335188db=ukj1871&indiv=try.

prepared by the trustees of the Seacole Fund, was extremely flattering, but highly inaccurate, with the same misinformation commonly given out by today's Seacole supporters. It says she learned nursing from her mother (who taught her traditional Creole herbals). She then 'greatly distinguished herself as a nurse on the battlefield and in hospitals during the Crimean War' (she did not nurse in any hospital during the war, but a few times gave first aid on the battlefield). It turned her stated intention to establish a 'mess table and comfortable quarters for sick and convalescent officers' into a reality. It exaggerated her presence 'at many battles' (she mentioned three in her memoir), and claimed that, 'at the risk of her life, often carried the wounded off the field' (she never described carrying anyone off the field, nor suggested that her life was at risk). It called her 'a patient nurse among those stricken with cholera,' without mentioning her use of mercury and lead in remedies. It quoted the warm tribute made by war correspondent W.H. Russell, but made him into a doctor. It correctly noted that the 'sum raised for Mrs Seacole enabled her to end her days in comfortable ease,' but incorrectly added that she bequeathed all her property to 'persons of title.'[88]

A letter to the editor soon after the obituary said that her sister was in 'straitened circumstances' in Jamaica and suggested that the 'persons of title' mentioned might assist her.[89] The writer, however, was misinformed, for Seacole left Louisa Grant, her main beneficiary, a significant £300 plus residuals, for an estimated total of £850, out of an estate valued at £2500. Their nephew Edward Ambleton, who was living in the smaller of Seacole's two houses, was left £100 and the house for life. Other relatives were given nineteen guineas, an odd sum which was Seacole's most frequent bequest. She left her old business partner, Thomas Day, the same nineteen guineas.

Bequests of £50 went to members of the Seacole Fund, as noted above in the sketches of her supporters. The president of the Legislative

---

[88] 'Obituary,' *The Times* 21 May 1881 7F.

[89] 'The Late Mrs Seacole,' *The Times* 24 May 1881 5B.

Council of Jamaica was left £50 and his daughter £200. Only one bequest went to a charity, £100 to the Cambridge Institution for Soldiers' Orphans. There is no mention of medals or testimonial letters in the will, although there are specifics for the disposition of her best bedstead and bedding, linen sheets, calico sheets, counterpane, other household linen, her watch, her husband's ring, other jewellery, trinkets and ornaments of the person, furniture, pictures, prints, engravings, plate and china.[90]

---

[90] Probate Office, will of Mary Seacole, 11 July 1881.

Chapter 4

The more prosaic adventures of
Ms Nightingale

Nightingale and the Crimean War

When the Crimean War began, Nightingale was superintendent of the
Establishment for Gentlewomen during Illness, in Upper Harley St.,
London, not the job she wanted, but at least she was nursing. Thanks to
stories in *The Times*, the terrible conditions suffered by the sick and
wounded were well known in Britain, as was the fact that the French had
women nurses, the Sisters of Charity, while the British did not.
Nightingale offered to go. She understood, as did her friends Sidney and
Elizabeth Herbert (he was the junior war secretary, she a member of the
ladies' committee at Harley St.), that this was her opportunity to realize
her calling from God.

Both Sidney and Elizabeth Herbert wrote her, he officially and at
great length,[1] while her short, heartfelt letter spoke to that calling.
Elizabeth told Nightingale that Sidney (clearly they were on a first-name
basis) would be writing the next day and assured her that leaving the
institution would cause no difficulties. The letter concluded:

> I can only say God guide you aright in your decision. I do feel that, if you
> refuse, you will have lost the most noble opportunity of doing the greatest

---

[1] Cook, *The Life of Florence Nightingale* 1:151–54.

possible amount of good, just *the* sort of good which *you* alone can do. We have plenty of hands offered, but no head, and the folly of some women is perfectly inconceivable....It is a great and national work to which you are called and it is God's work besides. I will say no more.[2]

Nightingale of course accepted and Mrs Herbert promptly wrote her again: 'My own dearest, noblest Flo, I *knew* you would do it and I am so impossibly thankful.' She was overly optimistic with her next remark: 'You will have seen Sid and every difficulty will be smoothed away.' She then went back to the calling:

> God be thanked that he has put his thought into your heart to go to do his work as you alone can. Sid longed to go to you last week, but he came down to consult me first and I persuaded him to write to you at once, as he did yesterday. But you really think of going tomorrow — it takes one's breath away.[3]

Not the least point of interest in this letter is that it shows the secretary of state at war consulting his wife on the appointment. The first-name familiarity does not reappear in the correspondence; all subsequent letters maintained the proprieties of 'Mr Herbert' and 'Miss Nightingale.'

When Nightingale led the first team of women to nurse for the British Army at war, she had minimal experience for the task at hand, although it was better than many later critics thought. Three months at Kaiserswerth taught her little about nursing, although she did at least have male patients, learned how to lay out the dead and got experience preparing drugs in the apothecary. She also spent some months in Paris hospitals, but what ward experience she had there is not clear. She observed operations conducted by an eminent surgeon, Professor Philibert-Joseph Roux, we know from later references.[4] Her administrative experience was confined to the small Harley St. institution. She only learned how to change dressings while at

---

[2] E. Herbert letter 15 October 1854, Claydon House bundle 289.

[3] E. Herbert letter 16 October [1854] Claydon House bundle 101.

[4] Nightingale remarked that she saw pyemia in his wards at the Hôpital de la Charité, Paris, letter 10 May 1862, in Lynn McDonald, ed., *Florence Nightingale and Hospital Reform* 575.

Scutari, from the experienced Mrs Roberts, who had nursed many years at St Thomas'. Nightingale herself recognized the greater administrative experience of the Rev Mother Mary Clare Moore, mother superior of the Sisters of Mercy at Bermondsey, who served under her. However, Moore had had no regular hospital experience.

During the war, Nightingale supervised the nursing at the Barrack Hospital at Scutari, the largest of all the British war hospitals, and at that point, the largest hospital in the world. She nursed and worked mightily behind the scenes to get supplies in, kitchens and laundries established and conditions improved. She was the 'general superintendent' of nursing in several other hospitals as well (each with its own local superintendent) and her administration was later extended to all the hospitals in the Crimea.[5]

Revealing stories in *The Times* on bad conditions and the lack of nursing in the Crimean War were instrumental to Nightingale being sent to the war in the first place. The paper then published occasional reports on her work and several letters to the editor she sent. Families who received letters from Nightingale on the death of their son sometimes sent them to the local newspaper and some to *The Times*.

On return from the war on 7 August 1856, Nightingale plunged into research to determine the causes of the high death rates. She kept a low profile. She visited Queen Victoria and Prince Albert at Balmoral Castle to discuss what became her 'confidential report' and pressed for the holding of a royal commission, which was duly appointed. The Royal Commission was chaired by Sidney Herbert, but she did much of the work for it from selecting the members and briefing witnesses to presenting her own evidence and analyzing data. The 'confidential report' Lord Panmure asked her to prepare was to have been a mere 'précis,' done in six months, but eventually became the 853-page *Notes on the Health of the British Army*. This work included material on civil hospitals

---

[5] For detailed coverage of her war work, see Lynn McDonald, ed., *Florence Nightingale: The Crimean War*.

as well and she soon had papers out on hospital reform per se, including both military and civil, for all hospitals had the same challenges with sanitation. The first paper, 'Notes on the Sanitary Condition of Hospitals, and on Defects in the Construction of Hospital Wards,' was given at meetings of the National Association for the Promotion of Social Science in 1858 and published in its *Transactions*. In 1863, she published a full book on hospital construction and administration, now with much new material, *Notes on Hospitals*.

In 1860, Nightingale published the first edition of her famous *Notes on Nursing*. Her nursing school at St Thomas' Hospital opened later that same year, financed by the Nightingale Fund, which had been raised in her honour during the war. That fund also paid for the midwifery training programme at King's College Hospital, which did not last, and for nurse training at several workhouse infirmaries, which did.

Nightingale, in short, was prodigiously active at research, policy determination and the introduction of nurse training and hospital reform right from her return from the war. She published a great deal. There was some, but only occasional, coverage of her in the popular press. She, like Seacole, visited army and navy hospitals post-Crimea, but Nightingale's visits were to see the physical plant with regard to sanitary conditions and arrangements for nursing and did not get press attention. However, the fact that she had visited the Melville Hospital and pronounced it to be 'the best of the national hospitals' was later relayed to the press by the duke of Somerset, first lord of the Admiralty.[6]

At the Scutari Barrack Hospital

An assistant to Lord Stratford de Redcliffe, British ambassador to Turkey, is a good source on Nightingale's work on first arriving at Scutari.

---

[6] 'Military and Naval Intelligence,' *The Times* 27 March 1857 10C.

From: James Henry Skene, *With Lord Stratford in the Crimean War* 37 and 38–39

Miss Nightingale had arrived here with her bevy of lady nurses. Her first act showed her wonderful energy and determination. The steamers laden with the wounded had cast anchor at Constantinople. There were not yet any mattresses or bedclothes on the camp beds in the hospital, and the latter were not nearly sufficient in number for the wounded coming. Miss Nightingale went to the quartermaster sergeant in charge of the stores and asked him for the stores which she required. He told her there was everything she could desire in the magazines, but that she must get the inspector general of hospitals to write an official letter to the quartermaster general, who would send him an authority to draw the stores and that she might then receive them on showing that authority. Miss Nightingale asked how long this would take. On being told that three days would be the shortest time necessary for the correspondence, she answered that 900 wounded officers and men would be in the hospital in three hours and that she must have what they required immediately. She then went to the magazines and, telling the sergeant of the guard there who she was, asked him if he would take an order from her. He said he would and she ordered him to drive in the door. This was done and the wounded were provided for in time.

Her firmness at surgical operations was something marvellous....She stood one day with spirits, instruments and lint in hand during the performing of a frightful amputation. Half a dozen young lady nurses were behind her, holding basins, towels and other things the surgeons might want. A harrowing groan from the patient suddenly put them all to flight, except Miss Nightingale, who, turning calmly round, called to them, 'Come back! shame on you as Christians! shame on you as women!' They returned holding each other's trembling hands, and some of them almost ready to faint. But they got over their nervous weakness...and did an amount of good that yet lives in the memory of many a man rescued from death and pain by their gentle ministrations.//

Lord Stratford's assistant also reported a wonderful anecdote of a commanding officer friend, who was a patient of Nightingale — there was some accommodation for officers at Scutari, which was mainly for ordinary soldiers.

From: James Henry Skene, *With Lord Stratford in the Crimean War* 120

> Another friend of mine...received a bad wound while going his rounds in the trenches, and had been conveyed to the hospital at Scutari, where Miss Nightingale nursed him. One morning he complained to her most bitterly of the noise which other wounded officers in the same ward had made in the night, having kept him awake when he wished to sleep. She told him that those officers had died in great agony. 'Well,' he said, 'I should feel so much obliged to you if, next time, you would ask any mortally wounded officers you may be taking care of in this ward to die quietly, without disturbing others in the night.' When I went to see him, he told me that Miss Nightingale had been wonderfully kind to him.//

He described his friend as the 'perfection of a commanding officer,' but with the defect of taking too much brandy (120–21). When he complained about the unhealthy climate of Constantinople, Skene remarked that he had never heard of it being unhealthy.

From: James Henry Skene, *With Lord Stratford in the Crimean War* 121

> 'Well,' he replied, 'all I can say is that I was not there a week before I had delirium tremens. I ought to have stayed at the hospital of Scutari, where Miss Nightingale assured me that neither she nor any of her lady nurses had ever had it. But I thought I had got so strong under their kind care that I should be proof against the infection of the delirium tremens, which is raging on the other side of the Bosphorus. The Greek patriarch and several of the ambassadors are suffering dreadfully from it. Constantinople has a bad climate, believe me.//

A Colonel Dawson, formerly of the 46th Regiment, reported the experience of a sergeant of his, Hampson, whom he left on the shore at Alma 'apparently dying,' who gave a good account of his treatment at Scutari in its early days.//

From: Michael Hargreave Mawson, ed., *Eyewitness in the Crimea* 59

> When he first went there, he was left...with several others in the hospital there in a room, and for seven days they never saw a doctor! He survived it, and says that now all is much better arranged. Miss Nightingale and her attendant angels he speaks most enthusiastically of. They were everywhere amongst the sick, doing more good than any doctors, and, as he somewhat naively observed, 'there was no sort of delicacy about them, Sir.'//

A useful early account comes from J.C. MacDonald, whose reports in *The Times* on the terrible conditions and lack of supplies were cited in Chapter 2. He arrived at Scutari at almost the same time as Nightingale and is likely the original source of the 'ministering angel' image. The item below reflects her early practice of walking through the wards alone late at night — later she had Private Robinson carry the lamp for her. In the example given here, the two patients she attended were doctors who died of fever.

From: Our own correspondent, 'The Sick and Wounded Fund,' *The Times* 8 February 1855 7E, dated 23 January 1855

> Both Newton and Struthers, it may be a consolation to their friends to know, were tended in their last moments, and had their dying eyes closed, by Miss Nightingale herself. Wherever there is disease in its most dangerous form and the hand of the spoiler distressingly nigh, there is that incomparable woman sure to be seen; her benignant presence is an influence for good comfort even amid the struggles of expiring nature. She is a 'ministering angel' without any exaggeration in these hospitals, and as her slender form glides quietly along each corridor, every poor fellow's face softens with gratitude at the sight of her. When all the medical officers have retired for the night, and silence and darkness have

settled down upon these miles of prostrate sick, she may be observed alone, with a little lamp in her hand, making her solitary rounds.//

On visiting the Koulali Hospital, Nightingale discovered that it had excellent bread, produced by the mission bakery which had initially supplied the Barrack Hospital, but whose contract was cancelled for failure to pay graft, as related in Chapter 2. As the next extract shows, she got the bread contract reinstated for Scutari, on better terms for the mission.

From: Cyrus Hamlin, *My Life and Times* 335 and 337

> Very soon Miss Nightingale transformed that hospital. From the first, she divided her forces into night watches, and there were nurses and assistant nurses walking those corridors and wards all night long. The nights were no longer lonely. Every want was attended to, every pain, if possible, assuaged.
>
> Her coming was soon after I had denounced the bread contract. She knew nothing of that until she visited the hospital at Koulali, where my bread was still used. She expressed surprise at such excellent bread, so superior to what she had at the great hospital. Dr Tice told her the whole story. She went immediately to Lord Stratford de Redcliffe and demanded that bread. He at once ordered my bread to be restored at the advanced price of the new contract.//

Nightingale did not keep a journal during the Crimean War, and, while hundreds of letters and notes by her survive, much yet is missing. A useful source to fill in some blanks is the memorandum written by Robert Robinson, a young Irish private who fell ill before the first battle was fought. He was sent to the Barrack Hospital in Scutari, where, on his recovery, he worked as a messenger and assistant to Nightingale. He wrote up these notes in 1860, at the request of a Nightingale relative. While the account is one of a devoted follower, it has the merit of reporting direct experience, both before and after Nightingale's arrival at the hospital. He became a protégé, working at the Nightingale family home after the war, and stayed in touch with Nightingale into his old age, as will be seen below in a letter of 1896.

From: Robinson memorandum, Add Mss 45797 ff83–85

[September 1854]

Nothing of importance occurred during the voyage until the morning of the 14th of September [1854] when we saw the Russian coast. In the afternoon of the same day, the armies landed without opposition. Throughout all these movements of the army I still remained with the 68th Regiment, and on the 14th of September I landed with my regiment on the Russian soil, but in the evening the doctor ordered me on board my ship again. From thence I was conveyed on board the *Kangaroo*, the first vessel that took sick from the Crimea.

The sight on board that vessel was something awful: 1300 sick and dying were packed on board this vessel, which was not fitted to carry 400. However, by the aid of another transport, the 1300 (minus thirty or forty who died on the passage) reached Constantinople on the morning of the 22nd of September. All the available hands were at once employed to assist in getting the sick ashore but, while doing so, the *Golden Fleece* came steaming down the Bosphorus with 300 or 400 wounded from the Battle of the Alma [20 September 1854]. It was a frightful sight to see some of the cases which came ashore on that day, and still more frightful to see them lying on stretchers in the passages of the hospital, and the men who were carrying them standing beside the stretcher, sometimes for two hours, waiting for orders where to take the man.

This was the weekly occurrence at the Scutari Hospital (for every week brought its sick from the Crimea) from September to November, and from that time onward everything underwent a change for the better. The sick were not kept waiting in the passages but went at once to bed, were washed and had clean linen and were attended as well as if in England.

All this, or the most part of it, was brought about by the influence and energy of a lady who had sacrificed every luxury at home to come out and administer comfort to her suffering countrymen. I think there were very few men of the many thousands who were sick at Scutari and the other hospitals in its neighbourhood who did not feel the comforting and beneficial influence of Miss Florence Nightingale. She went out with the intention to do good and that intention was carried out through every difficulty.//

War historian Kinglake's references to Nightingale were reverential, while he excoriated the army leaders for the deficiencies in the hospitals. If his praise was overly rambling and repetitive, it also contains some interesting comments on gender, in favour of the female sex which got things done, as opposed to the males running the War Office. The following excerpt conveys both the gruesome conditions and his esteem for Nightingale.

From: Alexander William Kinglake, 'The Winter Troubles,' *The Invasion of the Crimea* 6:425–26

There was worship almost in the gratitude of the prostrate sufferer who saw her glide into his ward, and, at last, approach his bedside. The magic of her power over men used often to be felt in the room — the dreaded, the blood-stained room — where 'operations' took place. There perhaps the maimed soldier, if not yet resigned to his fate, might at first be craving death rather than meet the knife of the surgeon, but when such a one looked and saw that the honoured lady-in-chief was patiently standing beside him, and — with lips closely set and hands folded — decreeing herself to go through the pain of witnessing pain, he used to fall into the mood for obeying her silent command, and, finding strange support in her presence, bring himself to submit and endure.//

Reform Club chef Alexis Soyer, who has been quoted in Chapter 3 on Seacole, provides much information on Nightingale at work. He had gone out to the war to introduce a whole new system of low-budget cooking, to provide nourishing, tasty meals within the limits of the soldiers' rations. His reforms were at first resisted, but Nightingale defended him. The memorandum by Private Robinson explained that, at first, Soyer 'was received but coolly by some of the authorities.' However, Nightingale 'stood his friend from the commencement and, by her influence, enabled him to carry out many of his plans, which otherwise he would not have been able to do.' He added that she saw the patients benefit 'from having their food cooked in a proper way, under the superintendence of such a skilful man of the art as M Soyer.'[7]

Soyer reported his first meeting with Nightingale at the Barrack Hospital in Scutari, where he found that the kitchen she had established there was the exception to the bad kitchens he had otherwise seen:

> We first visited Miss Nightingale's dietary kitchen, in which I immediately recognised the whole of the little camp batterie de cuisine which my friend Comte told me that the duke of Cambridge had presented to the hospital. Justice was indeed done to it, for every separate article of which it was composed was in use. Miss Nightingale had a civilian cook as well as an assistant. Everything appeared in as good order as could be expected (105).

He explained that 'a few days afterwards I closed all the extra diet kitchens with the exception of the one under the direction of Miss Nightingale and another under the direction of Dr Taylor' (134). Soyer and Nightingale worked together closely in the hospitals both in Scutari and later the Crimea to bring in the new system.

Soyer also recorded seeing Nightingale late at night in the wards, with her lamp, which he whimsically related in his memoir.

From: Alexis Soyer, *Culinary Campaign* 142–43

> As we turned the angle of the long corridor to the right, we perceived, at a great distance, a faint light flying from bed to bed, like a will-o'-the-wisp flickering in a meadow on a summer's eve, which at last rested upon one spot...But, alas! as we approached, we perceived our mistake. A group in the shape of a silhouette unfolded its outline in light shade. As we came nearer and nearer, the picture burst upon us. A dying soldier was half reclining upon his bed. Life, you could observe, was fast bidding him adieu....
>
> But stop! Near him was a guardian angel, sitting at the foot of his bed, and most devotedly engaged pencilling down his last wishes to

---

[7] Robinson memorandum, May 1860, Add Mss 45797 f98.

be despatched to his homely friends or relations. A watch and a few more trinkets were consigned to the care of the writer; a lighted lamp was held by another person [Private Robinson], and threw a painful yellowish coloris over that mournful picture, which a Rembrandt alone could have traced, but which everybody, as long as the world lasts, would have understood, felt and admired. It was then near 2 o'clock in the morning.

Approaching, I made inquiries of Miss Nightingale as to the complaint of her patient, when she replied, in French, that the poor fellow was given up by the doctors, and was not likely to get through the night, 'so I have been engaged noting down his last wishes, in order to forward them to his relatives.'//

In the Crimea

Nightingale made three visits to the Crimea during the war, the first in May 1855, when she soon came down with 'Crimean fever.' An army doctor reported upon her arrival that she was given a much better reception at Balaclava than she had at Scutari: 'Miss Nightingale has taken up her abode here, in a hut. She has been going over the various hospital establishments, where, of course, all the attention and respect she so well merits were paid to her.'[8]

A surgeon of the Light Infantry reported seeing Nightingale soon after her arrival in the Crimea.

From: Douglas Arthur Reid, *Memories of the Crimean War* 41

Not very long after Lord Raglan's visit, I was one day walking about the camp when I noticed a group of mounted officers, some evidently of high rank, approaching our lines. They turned out to be Lord

---

[8] Frederick Robinson, *Diary of the Crimean War* 314.

Raglan, General Pélissier [the French commander] and a number of staff officers, English and French, escorting Miss Florence Nightingale, who had come up from Scutari to see what provision had been made for the sick and wounded at the front. She visited the hospital, and I am afraid what she saw must have made her woman's heart bleed. But her visit was productive of much good. Through her report and her influence, the arrangements were improved and went on improving until the time came when, long before the war was over, we had almost a superabundance of medical comforts and even luxuries sent to the hospital.//

Nightingale's visit to another regimental hospital in early May was the subject of a letter by its surgeon, Ethelbert Blake, home to his wife, quoted in the next extract. He noted the 'incongruous party' approaching, including Nightingale, whom 'he had long wished to see.'

From: Christopher Hibbert, *The Destruction of Lord Raglan* 265

I was walking up and down the camp when we saw a lady and three gentlemen ride up to the hospital and an orderly came to say Miss Nightingale sent her compliments, to know if I had any objection to her going over my hospital. Of course I had none, so I joined the party, which consisted of Dr Sutherland (one of the Sanitary Commission), Soyer, and a half-caste!!![9] Miss Nightingale is a most pleasing person, refined and delicate, just fitted for the very trying position she fills. She was delighted with all she saw. x x Soyer was in raptures with my kitchen, built by Sergeant Desmore (the hospital sergeant) and, whilst Miss Nightingale and I were discussing matters of hospital detail, Soyer rushed up and carried her off to see the establishment, and his delight at the grate made of Turkoman gun barrels was beyond everything.//

---

[9] Soyer's secretary, Mr Taylor, a 'coloured gentleman,' according to Robinson's memorandum, below.

An officer of the 95th Regiment recalled the visit of Nightingale, with Soyer, to their camp and hospital, on 6 May 1855:

> Everyone turned out to see her, as all had heard of her good work in the Scutari hospital. Mr Alexis Soyer, the famous French cook, came at the same time and gave our men a lesson in cooking, showing them how to make the most of their rations. He certainly did make some most appetizing dishes, but the one lesson was not enough, and I do not remember that there was much improvement in the cooking in consequence.[10]

Nightingale would later get a cooking school established in the army to train soldiers to be cooks.

In addition to the space dedicated to work in the kitchens in his *Culinary Campaign*, Soyer recounted an excursion to a French lookout in the Crimea which he made with Nightingale and Dr Anderson, the principal medical officer. He evidently enjoyed the encounter, which he related with some humour, and which helps to give some context to the 'dangers' faced by the many visitors in the Crimea. He used the same term 'under fire,' clearly ironically, as Seacole did in her *Wonderful Adventures* (157).

From: Alexis Soyer, *Culinary Campaign*, 171–74

It was 4 o'clock and they were firing sharply on both sides... we formed a column and, for the first time, fearlessly faced the enemy and prepared to go under fire....The sentry begged of us to go into a kind of redoubt, built of stone, where there was a telescope. 'There,' said he, 'you will be in safety and have a good view of the town.'

This was true enough, the day being clear and the sun pouring its rays on the city, we could plainly discern the large buildings, Greek temple, church, club house, hospital, barracks, the harbour of Sebastopol and the fortifications, viz., the Malakhoff, Redan...and could see every shot sent by the allied armies as well as by the enemy. The bursting of shells could easily be distinguished. We

---

[10] John Richard Hume, *Reminiscences of the Crimean Campaign* 120–21.

were about to retire when Mr Anderson proposed going a couple of hundred yards further to the Three-Mortar Battery. Miss Nightingale immediately seconded the proposal, but the sentry strongly objected, saying it was too dangerous....

The sentry then repeated his caution, saying, 'Madam, even where you stand you are in great danger — some of the shots reach more than half a mile beyond this....Well, Madam, if you do not fear risking your life, I cannot prevent your going...I have witnesses to prove that it was not through my neglect in not informing you of the danger you incur by going to the Three-Mortar Battery.'

'My good young man,' replied Miss Nightingale in French, 'more dead and wounded have passed through my hands than I hope you will ever see in the battlefield during the whole of your military career. Believe me, I have no fear of death.'...

At all events, we arrived in the...battery without accident. It contained three large mortars...quite exposed to fire....We had, however, an excellent view of the besieged city, such as very few amateurs can boast of having obtained....

I then requested her to ascend the stone rampart next the wooden gun carriage and lastly to sit upon the centre mortar, to which requests she very gracefully and kindly acceded. I then boldly exclaimed, 'Gentlemen, behold this amiable lady sitting fearlessly upon that terrible instrument of war! Behold the heroic daughter of England — the soldier's friend!' All present shouted, 'Bravo!'...

At last we regained the redoubt, quite safe and sound, which the French corporal on duty attributed to their not thinking it worthwhile to fire upon us, and partly to the presence of a lady. He remarked that ladies often came to this spot to get a view, and that he had never known the enemy to fire while they were present.//

Private Robinson's memorandum, excerpted above, on Nightingale at Scutari describes travelling with her on her first trip to the Crimea. He reports on her falling ill, in the following excerpts.

From: Robinson memorandum, Add Mss 45797 ff87–89 and 92

The passage was a beautiful one of seventy-two hours. When the vessel got safe into Balaclava Harbour, Miss Nightingale thought about getting ashore, but as there was no place fit for her there, she agreed to remain on board the *Robert Lowe* as long as she stayed in harbour....

The day following...she, in company with Mr Bracebridge and M Soyer, visited the camp of the allies then before Sebastopol....

It was late in the evening when they returned, and Miss Nightingale seemed greatly overfatigued, as Mrs Roberts expressed it, 'quite done up,' and indeed she was done up, for the next morning I was despatched for the doctor, Dr Anderson, who was then the chief medical officer at the General Hospital. He attended immediately and threw us all into a state of alarm by saying he was afraid she had Crimean fever.

Further on in the day, several of the principal medical officers, Dr Anderson, Dr Hadley and Dr Sutherland, gave it as their joint opinion that she had fever of an alarming kind, and that, if possible, she should be removed from the ship to some healthy place on shore. On the following morning, she was carried by four soldiers on a stretcher from the London to the Castle Hospital on the heights near the Genoese Tower, where a hut was prepared for her reception.

It was a solemn procession. She who had administered comfort so many times to the sick should now need that comfort herself. She was accompanied from the ship to her hut on the hill by Dr Anderson, her attendant, Mrs Roberts, and a coloured gentleman (secretary to M Soyer), who held an umbrella in order to keep the sun's rays from the patient, and myself who walked behind, not strong enough to help to carry, nor tall enough to hold the umbrella....She was nursed there by one well qualified for the office, Mrs Roberts. For a fortnight we were all in uncertainty — she was so very ill and even the doctors had little hope of her recovery.

Time, which works wonders, wrought a change in Miss Nightingale, and slowly and surely she improved. When she became convalescent, an invitation was sent to her from the British Embassy at Constantinople to spend a few days at Therapia, on the shores of the Bosphorus, in order to gain her strength again. This she availed herself of, but only for a few days, for she was soon in the hospital again and at her work of doing good. During the time of her illness, I always brought little dainties that she could partake of from the hospital, as there was no kitchen in the house and everything had to be cooked at the hospital.//

According to Colonel Sir James Alexander, on Nightingale's first visit to the Crimea in 1855, she tried to get nurses established at the front, but the army thought the risks of mistreatment by their own troops too great. He had first seen her, 'a lady with a small party, among whom was Soyer,' riding past his hut. She was wearing 'a short and useful looking skirt...was of a good figure and ladylike, with a composed expression' (from the following extract, 2:158). When she was convalescing from Crimean fever, he went to visit her. The passage is of interest also in describing her attempt to devise a treatment for bedsores. Alexander was a supporter of the Inkermann Cafe and other measures to make life better for the ordinary soldier, as appears in the second excerpt.

From: James Edward Alexander, *Life of a Soldier, or Military Service in the East and West* 2:159–63

I rode one day with a medical friend, Dr P. Frazer KTS...to visit Miss Nightingale, 'the soldier's friend,' at the row of hospital huts below the old Genoese castle of Balaclava... Miss Nightingale's page, whom we met on the hillside above Balaclava, said his mistress was at home, and we found her in a clean room in a wooden hut which overlooked, with many others, the Black Sea; the grey towers of the castle of Balaclava were above them. Miss Nightingale had been suffering from fever — looked thin at this time, and was dressed in a bonnet, with a black dress and shawl. Spare white sheets on the walls formed a sort of tapestry to hide the boards; the table before her was covered with papers and work. She had visited the 14th hospital huts and approved of their condition, and she offered Dr Frazer, for the general hospital (to which he was attached), pillows with holes in them for bedsores.

Aware of the carelessness of some of the hospital orderlies, she was anxious to know if a supply of nurses would be of use in the front, but it was thought not safe to send them, for unless the huts were surrounded with palisades and shut off from the rest of the camp, the nurses might be interfered with.

One object of my visit to Miss Nightingale was to ask where we could get school books for the 14th Regiment; she promised some help, and I afterwards got a liberal supply of copy books from her and many numbers of the *British Workman* (monthly paper) which, with the Bible, were used as school books. We took leave much pleased with our visit, and, on the occasion of another visit, I had the satisfaction of seeing Miss Nightingale looking quite recovered, and well and cheerful. My countrywoman, Miss Shaw Stuart [Stewart], a coadjutor of Miss Nightingale in works of humanity and mercy, I also saw.//

Alexander reported that a school was duly established in a tent. Another tent was set up as a reading room with papers and odd volumes placed there, as well as games like skittles, quoits, rounders and nine holes. Means for bathing were provided 'by placing half a dozen half casks in a spare tent'; the casks were kept filled with water. A savings bank was started and money remitted home. He also noted that £60 was subscribed 'by all hands' to the Nightingale Fund, which, he said, was 'to raise a corps of army nurses,' which it was, partially, but it mostly supported civilian nursing (2:115).

Private Robinson's memorandum also covered Nightingale's second trip to the Crimea, in the autumn of 1855, which ended with her returning to Scutari to deal with a cholera epidemic.

From: Robinson memorandum, Add Mss 45797 ff92, 94 and 96–97

Having failed to carry out her good intentions on her first visit to the Crimea, she now meditated a second one, and, accordingly, on the 9th of October she repaired on board the first ship under orders for sailing (the *Ottawa*), accompanied by Mrs Roberts and myself.

This second visit was more hopeful than the first as Miss Nightingale enjoyed the best of health, and was able to carry out those projects which she anticipated doing on her first visit: one of these was the establishing of a staff of nurses at the Land Transport Hospital, which lay on the brow of an eminence looking down on that renowned plain where the great cavalry charge took place.

The commandant of the corps, Major, now Colonel, McMurdo was very anxious to have some of Miss Nightingale's influence in his hospital and gave her every assistance in his power. He sent two of his ambulance cars to convey the nurses from Balaclava.

When all things seemed settled satisfactorily...Miss Nightingale was requested by the medical men of the Monastery of St George's Hospital, if possible, to send some nurses to that place, as they were much needed. In order to distribute equally the benefit to all, and to comply with the request, she divided her staff at the General Hospital, Balaclava, and sent some of them under the superintendence of Miss Wear.

Having seen to all her arrangements [in the Crimea], and hearing that the cholera was making rapid strides at Scutari, she determined to proceed there at once. When she arrived, she was informed of the death of one of the principal medical officers, Dr McGrigor; he died of the disease and was deeply lamented by all, for he was one of the most energetic and clever men in the hospital....

During the time the disease was in its worst, Miss Nightingale made it her especial duty to attend on those cases and would not allow the other nurses to go near them. No matter where she was, she always had some especial patients of her own to look after, and those the worst cases in the hospital; for these she has often sat up until all others were asleep and with her little lamp (which I always trimmed) in her hand, I have many times seen her at 1 o'clock in the morning going her rounds, through the long passages and rooms of suffering in that ever-to-be-remembered Barrack Hospital. Many nights I have known her sit up all night with a patient and send the nurse, who should have sat up, to bed.//

Biographer E.T. Cook related a scene late in the war which nicely depicts the bureaucratic obstacles Nightingale continued to face, repeatedly, at the Barrack Hospital:

> On a cold night in January 1856, she was by the bedside of a dying patient whose feet she found to be stone cold. She requested an orderly to fetch a hot water bottle immediately. He refused, on the ground that his instructions were to do nothing for a patient without directions from a medical officer. Miss Nightingale stood corrected, and trudged off to find a doctor and make requisition for the bottle in due form.[11]

Letters from and about the Crimean War

Many Nightingale letters from the Crimean War have been published in a 1074-page volume in the *Collected Works of Florence Nightingale* and the collection cited in Chapter 2 by Goldie. Yet there are further letters of interest that are helpful in filling in the blanks that were not published in those sources. A selection appears here, in chronological order. The first letter shows Nightingale facilitating the use of chloroform (she brought supplies with her) at a time when the principal medical officer, Dr John Hall, opposed it. There are then two letters to her, typical of the requests for help she received. The first is from a sergeant at the hospital at Abydos, the second from a soldier's grandmother in England. After them come a variety of letters by Nightingale to her family and various other people, about hospital conditions and soldiers who died or disappeared. Subjects include the sad circumstances of a likely deserter, help for worthy hospital employees in later jobs and a testimonial letter for Soyer.

---

[11] Cook, *The Life of Florence Nightingale* 1:210.

From: Nightingale letter to an unnamed correspondent, Johns Hopkins University Medical Archives

Barrack Hospital, Scutari
10 December 1854

Would you take the trouble to find out and, if possible, procure an apparatus for the administration of chloroform, such as is used in the hospitals for operations, and send it me by the first opportunity, drawing upon our consul for payment.

Also, half a dozen of what in the French hospitals answer to our MacIntyre's or Liston's splints for compound fractures would be, if procurable, most acceptable here, and may be addressed to me. The sooner they can be had, the more acceptable.//

From: Two letters to Nightingale, Wellcome Trust RAMC 271/13 and /1 General Hospital

Abydos
7 January 1855

There are nearly 400 patients here who have been drafted periodically from Scutari as convalescents. These men are without either books or newspapers — have no money to buy stationery, which they much require, and many have not a change of linen.

Mr Stafford was here a few days since and, I believe, said in one of the wards that he would see and get those things remedied, but we understand he has gone to England and several of the men have expressed a wish that I would communicate with you on the subject.

This place is very lonely and, as in all other hospitals, the men cannot communicate with the world without. They are therefore altogether in the dark as to what is going on in the Crimea and in England, and if you will kindly cause a modicum of the papers sent from England by every mail to be redirected to this place you would confer a lasting obligation on us.

Dr Jameson, the principal medical officer here, is extremely kind to us and does everything in his power to make life tolerable in this out-of-the way place, but unfortunately he cannot supply us with newspapers or stationery, or I am sure he would.

With deep respect and gratitude I beg you will permit me to subscribe myself, Madam,

your obliged and very humble servant

G. Burden [sergeant of the 90th Foot Regiment]

25 January 1855

Your very benevolent feelings encourage me to hope you will excuse the liberty I take in addressing you and requesting you will, at your earliest leisure, give me an account of the death of George West, mentioned in this day's newspaper as having died on the 9th of January of dysentery, Ambulance Corps, at Scutari. Under any circumstances death always occasions melancholy feelings to the relations who are survivors, but it is more particularly painful to his mother, and myself as his grandmother — she having obtained for him a cadetship to India — and was with a tutor and nearly passed his first examination for the appointment when suddenly he started off and placed himself in the 46th Regiment....

I pray you to let us know as full particulars as possible, if any communications were made for us and if his sufferings were great, if any clergyman was with him, and, in short, all that you can possibly collect of information that you know will be a comfort to us....

With every good wish for your health, as regards yourself and those you have so nobly undertaken to comfort, and believe me I am, dear Madam,

yours with my sincere respect

Laetitia Elizabeth Prescott//

From: Nightingale letter to her mother, Frances Nightingale, Wellcome Trust Ms 8995/3

Scutari Hospitals

1 February 1855

We have no cholera. Your mind seems sorely troubled about chloride of lime [a bleach]. Can you suppose that such a scavenger as I am have not a sack of chloride of lime at the corner of every corridor and do not myself see to the fatigue parties cleansing out the places which require it? Alas! I am purveyor, scavenger, everything to these colossal calamities, as the hospitals of Scutari will come to be called in history.

I do read your letters. I do not read *The Times*.

ever yours, dearest people, which means a great deal, I assure you, in a place where envies and emulations and official jealousies interfere with the lives of men.

F. Nightingale

S. Herbert has borne me out gallantly on Commissariat reforms.//

From: A copy of a Nightingale letter to her family, Wellcome Trust Ms 8995/8

Scutari

5 March 1855

Dearest people

I saw Athena last night. She came to see me. I was walking home late from the General Hospital round the cliff, my favourite way, and looking, I really believe for the first time, at the view: the sea glassy calm and of the purest sapphire blue, the sky one dark deep blue, one solitary bright star rising above Constantinople, our whole fleet standing with sails idly spread to catch the breeze, which was none...a large fleet of Sardinians carrying up Sardinian troops, the domes and minarets of Constantinople sharply standing out against the bright gold of the sunset, the transparent opal of the distant hills (a colour one never sees but in the East), which stretch below Olympus, always snowy, and on the other side the Sea of Marmora, when Athena came along the cliff quite to my feet, rose upon her tiptoes, bowed several times, made her long melancholy cry and fled away — like the shade of Ajax. I assure you my tears followed her.

On Wednesday February 28th we had the sharp shock of an earthquake. It is indescribable. One does not feel the least frightened, but I felt quite convinced our old tower must come down. 200 patients jumped out of bed and ran into the main guard. Two jumped out of window. Some got out of bed who could not get in again. When next we looked across to the other side, two minarets of Constantinople had disappeared. Half Bursa is in ruins, and the accounts of killed and wounded there, where statistics are none, vary from 3,000 to 800. One man here with a compound fracture seriously injured himself by scuttling out of bed. We have had several slight shocks since.

    ever yours

    F.N.//

Athena, in the above letter, was the owl Nightingale rescued from boys who were tormenting it when she visited the Parthenon in 1850. She took it back to England with her, but it died on her departure for the East in October 1854. The earthquake referred to later in the letter was severe — magnitude 7.5 on the Richter scale.

From: 'Letter from Miss Nightingale,' *The Times* 29 September 1855 7E

Scutari, Barrack Hospital

18 August [1855]

Dear Mrs [blanked out]

    I very much regret to be obliged to inform you that your husband [blanked out] of the Artillery, was brought in here sick of diarrhea, with symptoms of fever, on the 11th of August from the Crimea.

    He asked me for a religious book, and I gave him the enclosed. He told me afterwards that he liked it very much, and so I send it to you, with another which he was already reading, a New Testament, and a letter of yours which was under his pillow, and his purse, containing £1.1.

    He was taken worse on the 13th and became delirious. He was most carefully attended by two doctors, by the chaplain, by myself and by a kind and skillful nurse. He was very grateful and good, but alas! nothing could save him and he died at 11 o'clock the same night. How sorry I am to tell you this bad news I cannot say.

    From the little I saw of your husband, I should say that his was a heart turned to God, and accepted by him. Let us hope that what is your loss is his gain. He often spoke of you. Believe me,

    yours with true sympathy

    Florence Nightingale//

From: An incomplete letter probably to her aunt, Mai Smith, Wellcome Trust Ms 8995/59

Castle Hospital
Balaclava
29 October 1855

Could you delicately say to Miss Clarke that the newspapers have not, in any one single instance, come right? If she has distributed the others in the same way, there must have been grievous disappointments. Sometimes there comes one old and one new one — sometimes the newest one not at all, but two duplicates of the old, etc. As soon as the papers arrive, she must (or you will be so good, please, as to) make up the new sets to go, and never mix them afterwards. There is nothing but his rum, alas! that a soldier cares about so much as his newspaper....Many thanks.//

From: Nightingale draft letter for the family of a soldier, Wellcome Trust Ms 8995/73

Castle Hospital
Balaclava
12 November 1855

Thomas Parr, late private of the 28th Regiment, well remembered by Lt and Adjutant H.C. Worthington, both recruits at drill together at Newcastle-on-Tyne in 1853. He was a good soldier to his country and, it may be said, to his Saviour also.

Please tell this to his family. I announced his attested death to you in my last.//

From: Nightingale letter to her family, Wellcome Trust Ms 8995/74

Castle Hospital
Balaclava
14 November 1855

The camp gossip here is that the Codrington appointment [as commander of the Light Division] is only a warming pan — and that General Wyndham [Windham], chief of the staff, is to have the honour of next year's campaign at Nicholaieff, with the command-in-chief. Though the whole camp is as cautious as Ladies of the Bedchamber, none scruple now to say, General Simpson being gone, that the whole failure of the Redan rests with him — that, had the Highland Brigade, with the Third Division to support them, led the attack, we could not have failed, with the loss indeed of three times the men to have carried the Redan and all before us, taken the little Redan and the Russian Army in flank and all but annihilated it.

Sir John Hall is going back to his rupees in India [his previous appointment was in India] with a KCB ship [Knight Commander of the Bath]. It is like the lifting off of a great incubus [evil spirit], and everybody seems to breath more freely. Now I think something may be done in the Crimea — I feel as if my hands were untied. Dr Hall's probable departure makes my stay here as long as the war much more certain. I do not think he would ever have made me desert my post — nor by rendering what I could do little, make me give up the little I could do. But, though I hope experience has long since caused me to cease either to hope or to fear, but simply to act and to trust, I do, though I may be most excessively mistaken, expect great reforms from the absence of this incubus.

The dirt he has walked through in opposing and thinking to sting me is wonderful — for he really is an able and efficient officer — with a head square like Napoleon's and as vain — as inclined to dirty tricks as that great ruffian. Dr Hall has actually stooped, as I know from authority that cannot be doubted, to tell the nurses I have sent to the Crimea that they may take off their badges, that they may cease to consider themselves as under my authority and that he will provide if they will desert me — he will pay them.//

From: A copy of a Nightingale letter, Florence Nightingale Museum

Castle Hospital

Balaclava

21 November 1855

Sir [Agent of Transports]

An outbreak of cholera at Scutari renders my return there urgently desirable.

I learn that the *Indiana* sails today. Could you grant passages upon her for myself, one nurse and a boy as far as Scutari? You will oblige me most exceedingly.

Will you let me know the latest hour of her sailing?//

From: Report on nurses, Wellcome Trust Ms 8995/78

[December 1855]

It will also be shown that the mortality in the female staff has been, during the above period, rather less than 6 percent, the total loss from sickness and death rather less than one fourth.

Comparing this with the mortality and invaliding among the medical officers, chaplains, etc., of the Army in the East, the proportion will appear to be comparatively small — although the exposure to infection and to the influences of disease is, obviously, greater among nurses. This comparative immunity may probably be attributed to the simplicity and regularity of habits enforced among them (this very small proportion arises from the too great haste in the selection)....

It will be seen that the proportion of those sent home (from every cause) is 64/108. It may, therefore, be inferred that the female staff will require renewing about every two years for the following reasons:

1. on account of the climate and other causes of disease;

2. because intoxication, tacitly admitted as unavoidable among nurses in London hospitals, must, in military hospitals, be sternly checked, by dismissal at the first offence, in order to carry on the work at all;

3. because, with every care exercised in the selection (which unfortunately has not always been the case) a certain proportion of incompetents or adventurers, tempted by high pay, by vanity or curiosity, or because they cannot live at home, will always be amongst those sent out;

4. because women, as well as men, will fall homesick at the end of one or two years, and are then of little use to the queen's service. But, taking all these drawbacks into consideration, which apply (not more but perhaps) less to the female than to any other branch of the service, it is obvious that the experiment of sending nurses to the East has been eminently successful, and that the supplying trained instruments to the hands of the medical officers has saved much valuable life and remedied many deficiencies.//

From: A copy of a Nightingale letter probably to her mother, Frances Nightingale, Wellcome Trust Ms 8995/82

[ca. December 1855]

I send by Mr Cooper, steward of *Indiana*, 1 box with the vines in it from our vineyard at the Castle Hospital (I am told that the way they are cut, though not your way, is the only way that would do); 1 Russian sword cartridge, as my portion of Sebastopol spoil to be sent to my warlike father; 1 Russian cap, Robert's, to be sent to his mother, Mary Robinson, care of Mr J. Stewart, 12 Cullingtree St., Belfast, as his portion of Russian spoil....

Would you desire all these things to be called for and distribute them accordingly. Robert is going to send you a sword all to yourself.

I was brought back suddenly from Balaclava by the cholera here. [Dr] McGrigor is dead and four other surgeons whom you don't know — deaths just under half the operation cases — subsiding now rapidly. German Legion moved out of this hospital in consequence...

Any quantity of books which can be sent out is acceptable. Remember we are 50,000.//

137

From: Nightingale letter to Colonel Gordon Drummond, Christie's sale list

> General Hospital
> Balaclava
> 15 April 1856

Sir

May I venture, although a stranger to you, to apply to you upon a matter which is of some importance to our hospitals?

Samuel Vickery, a private in the Coldstreams under your command, was frostbitten soon after Inkermann, and sent down to hospital at Scutari. He recovered sufficiently to become one of my orderlies, though not to rejoin his regiment.

This man has, during sixteen months, cooked the extras (for the patients) in my Extra Diet Kitchens, assisted me materially in the stores, and, by his diligence, sobriety, trustworthiness and cleverness, made himself of essential [use].... On one occasion he was the principal means of discovering a robbery of a large amount of stores.//

From: Nightingale letter to the sister of a soldier, University of Chester

> General Hospital
> Balaclava
> 20 May 1856

Madam

It is with sincere sorrow that I am obliged to confirm the fears of the father of the late Howell Evans about his poor son.

I grieve to say that Gunner and Driver Howell Evans, of the No. 1 Company, 12th Battalion, Royal Artillery, was struck off the strength of this Army 29 June 1855 as having been 'missing since 5 February 1855.' His company was in the siege train and went home in February 1856. It is now at Woolwich. His father had better apply at the Office of the 12th Battalion — no trace of the missing man being obtainable here.

To you, Madam, I will say that, after the most diligent inquiry, it appears to the commanding officer of the unfortunate man, and to myself, from the evidence, to be feared that Howell Evans is a deserter.

To the father I would say (if, on inquiry at the above address it appears that nothing more is to be learnt) that I regret very much that I am unable to send him any of those particulars concerning his son which it is natural that he should wish to hear, but, though I have made every inquiry in my power, I am unable to do more than send him the sad certainty of his death (for I would fain put it so).

Although it be impossible to us to retain particulars of the deaths of all those brave soldiers who have died in the service of their country during that fearful winter, it is a comfort to me, who have seen so much of their patient suffering, to remember that no one is forgotten by the Father of us all. I trust it will be a comfort to the father to remember that all are in his hands.

I doubt not he has suffered much from painful uncertainty concerning his poor son. Let him (if no further news is obtained) know that he now is at rest from all cares and sorrows of this world. May he be supported to bear them till it please God that those who have been separated by death will meet again in the better life to come.

I have never had so painful and unsatisfactory a letter to write. I beg to remain, Madam,

> your obedient servant
> Florence Nightingale//

From: Nightingale letter to an unknown officer, Bodleian Library ff279–80

> General Hospital
> Balaclava
> 23 June 1856

My dear Sir

1. Would it be possible to send six Commissariat casks to Mrs Shaw Stewart, Left Wing Hospital, Land Transport Corps, of those you kindly offered me?

2. Could you inform me how I could send to the Russian hospitals certain stores which might be useful to the Sisters of Charity?

3. I think there is no occasion for me to look at the *Spartan*'s berths. I shall occupy the six to Scutari which you have been so kind as to offer me, and for so short a distance, I shall not separate my commissioned and non-commissioned nurses on board.

4. I will ask you to remember my seven left behind about whom I am anxious, as I am compelled myself to return to Scutari without waiting to pack them off.

I enclose a letter from Lord Panmure, which I presume he wrote to meet an exigency like the present. I am sure that you will know that I do so — not to make public the flummery which he there vouchsafes to us women, who have merely done our duty as hospital nurses — but to show you that we are not on the same footing as the officers' wives who have come up here to amuse themselves, and who are obliged to ask for passages as a favour. I have steadily refused to bring up one woman here except on duty.//

From: A copy of a letter to the mother of a soldier, Wellcome Trust, Phillips catalogue 13/3/97

Barrack Hospital
Scutari
28 July 1856

I have seen your son and spoken to him on the subject of your letter. He tells me that he has written to you several times through his grandmother. He has also sent you £10. x x

I can give you a very satisfactory account of your son — he has been made not only a corporal, but sergeant. He is in very good health and is, I believe, conducting himself very well. x x [He] sends condolences x x . Your son has received all your letters and was aware of his poor sister's death. He is much attached to you, as I can see by what he says.//

From: Nightingale testimonial letter, in Soyer, Culinary Campaign 417

> Scutari
> Barrack Hospital
> 28 July 1856

I have great pleasure in bearing my testimony to the very essential usefulness of Monsieur Soyer, who, first in the general hospitals of Scutari, and afterwards in the camp hospitals of the Crimea, both general and regimental, restored order where all was unavoidable confusion, as far as he was individually able, took the soldiers' rations and patients' diets as they were, and converted them into wholesome and agreeable food.

I have tried his stoves in the Crimean hospitals where I have been employed and found them answer every purpose of economy and efficiency.//

Post-war, Nightingale back in England

On her return to London, Nightingale continued to respond to requests for help on particular persons, while her main work devolved to ascertaining what went wrong in the war hospitals and what to do differently in the future. An example of the former shows her trying to determine the whereabouts of a missing son of a Derbyshire neighbour and family friend, Mrs Hurt of Alderwasley Hall. Mrs Hurt had lost two sons in the war, one from wounds at the Battle of Inkermann, who was buried on Cathcart's Hill, while the other presumably died on the first Redan assault of 18 June 1855, but his body was never found.

Nightingale saw that Mrs Hurt 'seemed still suffering from the idea that she might have heard more about her two great griefs and the circumstances attending them.' She had seen this in other 'poor mothers' and tried her best to provide information for them. She found the names and addresses of officers who had last seen the missing son and the assistant surgeon who had sat up with the son wounded at Inkermann.[12]

The letter following responds to the same desperate request for help, this time with a possible happy outcome. The letter following it shows Nightingale pursuing a very different matter, the annual cost of a soldier.

From: Nightingale letter to family on a soldier's disappearance, private collection

London

2 November 1856

Dear Madam

I was quite puzzled by your letter of 10 September. I feel so deeply for the mothers whose uncertainty regarding the fate of their sons during the late war I have always felt it my duty to take every pains to relieve that.

I caused again a search to be made in our Death Books for the man's name in question. Inspector-General Linton reports to me as follows: 30 October 1856, 'It appears from the Death Book at the office that No. 2899, Private William Wood of the 2nd Battalion Rifle Brigade, died of erysipelas on the 14th of February 1855 — but, as the name of Private William Wood of the 1st Battalion Rifle Brigade does not appear in the books as having been admitted into the Scutari hospitals after Inkermann, there is every probability that this man is serving with his battalion.'

I give you the extract verbatim. You will observe the difference between 1st and 2nd Battalion, and that the name has not the final s. I should be very glad if I could think that the son of your dear old nurse was yet living. You will but know the precision of the information you have received from the War Department. I have known alas! upwards of 1,600 unreported deaths. Believe me to be, dear Madam,

yours faithfully

Florence Nightingale//

---

[12] Nightingale letter 17 November 1856, Private collection, Derbyshire.

From: Nightingale letter to T. Graham Balfour, army statistician, Staffordshire County Council, Lichfield Record Office

23 April 1858

Dear Dr Balfour

Dr Sutherland understood you to say yesterday that in General Lawrence's evidence in your report, I should find an estimate of the annual cost of the soldier. I cannot. And I dare say he made a mistake. Could you tell me the page where it is to be found?//

The next letter below shows Nightingale analyzing the consequences of what she considered Raglan's fatal appointment of Dr Andrew Smith as head of the Army Medical Department. The correspondence referred to shows medical officers in the field reporting terrible lacks, and the non-response or inadequate response by the department in meeting them. The appendix was only published in the second volume of the Royal Commission Report, by which time Nightingale had her 'confidential report' printed and ready for release. However, she considered the contents so important — the letters showed precisely who knew what when, but failed to act — that she added whole new sections quoting them to her own report. This made her report bulky and confusing to follow, for the new sections and pages were given Roman numerals. However, the inclusion of this material enabled her to be even tougher and more precise in her analysis.

In a letter to her sister, the second below, Nightingale had cause to remember the personnel of the Sanitary Commission that had done the work on the ground that reduced the death rates.

From: Nightingale letter to Sidney Herbert, Wiltshire County Record Office, Pembroke Collection 2057/F4/67

24 October 1858

I don't know whether you will think it wise to look back to the old Crimean story. But the height of absurdity in that correspondence (of Appendix LXXIX of your report) has never been surpassed. You might treat it à la Rabelais in your article.

What was the practical result of all that bulk of letters? The sending out of lime juice, which was not distributed till too late, and of peat charcoal, which was not wanted. This was all.

What can one say more in condemnation of a department? What was it there for? There is nothing in Molière to compare with this.

Lord Raglan was the primary cause of [Andrew] Smith's appointment. Never perhaps was a more fatal act committed by a more honest man. It cost him his army and his reputation. If you, as an administrator, were to touch it up, as you well know how, so as to extract the ha'porth of bread out of all that abominable deal of sack, I think it might do good.//

From: Nightingale letter to her sister, Parthenope Verney, Wellcome Trust (Claydon copy) Ms 8997/79

26 October 1858

Pray thank Sir Harry very much for his very kind note about Liverpool, and say that I remember the two men, Freeney and Aynsley, perfectly, and was very glad to hear they remembered me. They and another (Wilson, who was my particular friend) were the three inspectors of nuisances in the Crimea and at Scutari (Aynsley and Freeney in the Crimea and Wilson at Scutari) and were much more useful men than Airey, Gordon and Estcourt[13] or any of that genus. Lord Shaftesbury sent out the whole concern, under a civil engineer of Liverpool (Newlands) and they cleaned away at us right well. (Sutherland and Rawlinson were the heads of the commission.)//

---

[13] Sir Richard Airey was the quartermaster general, Colonel Gordon his assistant, Major General Estcourt the adjutant general — all implicated in the failure of supplies.

From: A copy of a Nightingale letter to an unknown person, Wellcome Trust sale catalogue 1332 (2005)

22 November 1858

My dear Sir

It is an old story now. The interest of the Crimean War, as a narrative, has passed away to most people. And it is only the general application — of which above all others, this war is capable, to universal sanitary relations — that I think will interest you.

The report is really 'confidential,' has not been laid on the table of the House of Commons, and is in no sense a public document and I must, therefore, ask you not to let it be on your table nor to let anyone else read it.//

From: Nightingale letter to John Arthur Roebuck, MP, British Library RP 7945 (I)

23 November 1858

Sir

In venturing to send you a copy of the Report to the War Office, I am encouraged to do so, not by any hope that you will remember me, but by the great public services which you rendered at the time of the Crimean disaster of which it treats.

That is an old story now. But the great sanitary interests of the army to which it refers are never old. Nor are the good sense, the heroic simplicity and the indomitable patience of our men, which are there recorded.

I do not conceive that you will have leisure or inclination to read this report yourself. But I am obliged to request that you will not let anyone else read it, as it is in no sense a public document.//

Nightingale continued to be exasperated with the complacency and inefficiency of the War Office after the war. The Royal Commission gave its well-crafted recommendations in 1858, but getting them implemented so as to save lives was an ongoing struggle. In the 1860 letter below she complained to Sidney Herbert about the same problems she had encountered during the war.

From: Nightingale letter to Sidney Herbert, Wiltshire County Record Office 2057/F4/68

3 September 1860

People talk of my 'terrible and unprecedented experience of the inefficiency' in the Crimea — I say my 'terrible and extraordinary experience of the inefficiency' in the War Office during the last four years. No one would believe it who had not seen it. The intentions of the secretary of state are no more carried out than if he were at Timbuctoo.

The
1. slowness
2. inefficiency
3. extravagance in administration
4. want of unity
are beyond all belief.//

Nightingale mostly avoided making judgments that were properly the province of medicine, but she did occasionally comment on such matters. In her 1858 *Notes on the Health of the British Army*, she faulted the Army Medical Department for failing to make 'any remarks as to the caution required in prescribing remedies such as calomel' (*CW* 610). In a letter to sanitary expert Edwin Chadwick, she noted that people took 'water cures' to get the mercury out of their system. In a letter to Sidney Herbert, she referred to 'quack physicians' using calomel.[14]

Calomel was then commonly deployed — it was available without prescription — as a home-remedy purgative. It was widely used as well by doctors, in many countries. Lead acetate similarly was widely used as a remedy. Nightingale is not known to have used or advised the use of either. The term 'lead acetate' does not appear in her writing and mercury (calomel) appears only when she is deriding its use.

---

[14] Letters to Edwin Chadwick 16 September 1860, Add Mss 45770 ff182–83 and to Sidney Herbert 8 June 1861, Wiltshire County Record Office 2057/F4/69.

The last two letters show Nightingale following up on people she knew during the war who later needed help, in the first case, a doctor's widow.

From: Nightingale letter to Captain E. Gardiner Fishbourne, Royal Navy, Add Mss 45800 f229

12 February 1868

If anything can be done for Mrs George Taylor's case, as enclosed, under the amended act, I am sure that the commissioners will take it under their favourable consideration.

I knew Dr George Taylor very well. I shall never forget how he worked at the difficult task of organizing the Medical Service of the Land Transport Corps in the Crimea War. After he had put it in order, I went up from Scutari by order and took over the female nursing of the two hospitals of the Land Transport Corps under him in the Crimea. I knew much of his exertions and able, willing conduct of a very severe task from beginning to end. I should be much pleased if anything could be done for the family of so zealous and wise a public servant as was Dr George Taylor.//

Nightingale wrote the next letter on the death of her friend and colleague, Dr John Sutherland, whom she first met when he arrived in Scutari at the head of the Sanitary Commission. In identifying herself as 'his pupil,' she recognized his critical importance in her own development as a public health reformer. The key principles she used, which would now be called 'evidence-based health care,' she learned from him. The obituary published two days later would seem to be hers, or at least partly hers. It tellingly ends with the statement that the value of his work could be seen 'by a comparison between the vital statistics of the army prior to the time of the Crimean War and those of the present date.'[15]

The last letter goes back to the messenger, Private Robert Robinson, who carried the lamp for Nightingale after his recovery at the Barrack

---

[15] Obituary, *The Times* 24 July 1891 8D.

Hospital early in 1855. She got him out of the army and into school. He became a landscape gardener and she helped him find jobs. A few cordial letters from him show he kept in touch. She occasionally sent him money and left him £175 in her will.[16] This letter was to Sir Harry Verney's son — Sir Harry had previously assisted Robinson, who had married a local woman, in getting another position. However, the excerpted section is on Crimean days.

From: Nightingale letter to the editor of *The Times*, TNL Archive PHL/2/221

22 July 1891

Private.

Though unwilling to trespass upon your attention, may I say that it would give me infinite pleasure if you are able to insert in your world-circulated paper the notice of Dr Sutherland, the great sanitarian, which I understand was sent you this morning with a note from Dr Marston.

I was associated with Dr Sutherland in his sanitary labours, not only in the Crimean and Scutari hospitals, but also in the fourteen successive years after our return from the Crimean War. I may say I was his pupil both in sanitary administration and practice, and am anxious for my master's fame.

May this serve as my apology for troubling you?//

From: Nightingale letter to Frederick Verney, Add Mss 68888 ff164–65

9 February 1896

But I can speak for R.R. as one can speak for few — though not professionally. I have known him for forty-one years, beginning in the Crimea where I could trust him to buy things for the patients on board

---

[16] For example her cheque for £5 in 1888 in the London Metropolitan Archives H1/ST/NC18/21/58; his letter in 1894, in H1/ST/NC2/V1/94; her will in Lynn McDonald, ed., *Florence Nightingale: An Introduction to her Life and Family* 854.

the ships at Balaclava (and never drink) as I could trust no man. He was then sixteen — I bought him out of the army, educated him....

R.R. married a Claydon girl.... He has never made a faux pas. When I saw him the other day, he was still the same upright, open, little fellow he was forty-one years ago. There is something that a good young soldier never loses.//

Nightingale's research and writing on the Crimean War

After the war, Nightingale's work on preventing its high death rates from recurring began in earnest. Her lengthy *Notes on the Health of the British Army* and the much shorter 'Answers to Written Questions' were major pieces of research. 'Answers to Written Questions' was her written evidence given to the Royal Commission, probably to questions which she herself requested to be asked. Her answers range from short and pithy to long and data laden. To the question 'To what do you mainly ascribe the mortality in the hospitals?' she gave a three word answer: 'To sanitary defects' (Question 22, in *CW* 902).

In answer to Question 25 on how 'the sanitary conditions of the soldiers before and after 17 March 1855 differed from the sanitary conditions of patients in civil hospitals,' she highlighted the work of the Sanitary Commission. After it, she concluded, 'I know no buildings in the world which I could compare with them,' still excepting 'the original defects of construction' (*CW* 912). She expanded on the defects in answering Question 26, wondering rhetorically about the high mortality, and why it was not worse, given the conditions. She described the faulty privies which 'poured their poisons into the corridors and wards, the sewers being loaded up with filth,' a code word for feces. For several months in that first winter the privy was 'too horrible to describe,' with its inch deep of 'filth.' The drinking water had 'organic matter' in it, which included, but was not confined to, fecal material. As bedpans were lacking, tubs were put into the wards, which she got emptied. The burial of the dead resulted in further pollution. After detailing these, and other, defects, she noted the rise in mortality on cases treated from 17.9 % in December, to 32.1 % in January and 42.7 % in February, although by February the hospitals were not so badly overcrowded and the cases coming to them were not so bad: 'What else could this increase be due to but to our defective sanitary condition?' (*CW* 913–14).

For her lengthier *Notes on the Health of the British Army*, Nightingale drew on the reports of the investigative commissions, especially the Sanitary Commission, and brought in much comparative material on civil hospitals. She set out causes (five) for the high mortality at Scutari: overcrowding, inadequacies in ventilation, drainage, cleanliness (especially washing), and medical comforts (bad cooking, inadequate food distribution, lack of utensils for eating, and lack of shirts and sheets), on each of which she produced pages of evidence (*CW* 732). She gave other lists of causes as well, all of them multiple. For the high death rate in Bulgaria before a shot was fired, she cited 'the unhealthy nature of the ground, want of proper food, of proper clothing, of shelter from the sun and of medical supplies' (*CW* 612). Later in the report she listed the conditions a medical officer should look at when infectious diseases appeared: defective drainage, overcrowding, defective ventilation, want of cleansing, nuisances, unburied animals, bad water, food, defective clothing, exposure or fatigue, and damp or wet ground (*CW* 666).

Nightingale also devoted considerable energy and space to showing how slow the Army Medical Department in London was to act when doctors sent in reports of the desperate conditions and missing necessities. She excerpted a letter by Dr Andrew Smith, director general of the Army Medical Department, ordering a clean-up, written on 9 March 1855. This was three days after the Sanitary Commission had started making the drastic changes needed. He could have and should have ordered the work done earlier, she thought. His letter pointed out 'the most prominent of those sanitary defects, which had converted these hospitals into pest houses.'

But why so late? Why did he delay writing so long? Was there no medical officer who could have told Dr Smith, before the hospitals were occupied, that they were not ventilated and that the sewers 'discharged their gases into the buildings,' a fact which was as true before they were occupied with sick as it was when Dr Smith wrote?

The result was that sick men went to the hospitals 'in the hope of life,' but were 'sacrificed to the utter want of sanitary knowledge or system in the department.' The clean-up was not accomplished until April 1855, but the defects were noted early in the war: 'The greater part of these nuisances had been reported on by and to the then principal medical officer as early as May 1854' (*CW* 645). Learning about defects in a timely manner would be a concern of Nightingale's to the end of her working life.

With the benefit of hindsight, it is clear that the Crimean War was formative for Nightingale. Not only did the funds raised in her honour permit the founding of her nursing school, the first in the world, she would apply the methodology she learned from analysing what went wrong to her research from then on. The careful attention she paid to getting the right person for any hospital or nursing appointment or government commission, and the necessity of starting small and checking results before generalizing, came out of that early work. So also did her insistence on careful ongoing monitoring of any new programmes or treatments that stem from the war experience.

Chapter 5

The myths exposed

*'For the time is coming when people will not put up with sound doctrine, but, having
itching ears, they will accumulate for themselves teachers to suit their own desires, and will
turn away from listening to the truth and wander away to myths'*
(St Paul, 2 Timothy 2–4)

*'It often falls out that somewhat is produced of nothing, for lies are sufficient to breed
opinion, and opinion brings on substance'*
(Francis Bacon, 'Of Vainglory,' Essays, Civil and Moral No. 14)

The biographical sketch of Mary Seacole in Chapter 3 bears little
resemblance to the person who emerges here, the mythologized Seacole of
the *Nursing Standard*, the BBC, the UK Department of Health, the Seacole
Memorial Statue Campaign and its supporters, many websites and social
media. Transformed from a plucky, generous businesswoman and herbalist,
Seacole has been recreated as a professional nurse, nurse practitioner, or
even a doctor, an organizer of professional nursing services and hospitals, a
war heroine and frequent daredevil on the battlefield where she even
treated the sick — whatever were the sick doing on the battlefield?

No fewer than ten distinct myths have evolved to create this
mythologized version of Mary Seacole. Four relate her feats during the
Crimean War, which is where we will start. Three others concern nursing
and there is one each on her volunteering to go to the Indian mutiny, race

issues and her relationship with Nightingale. They are refuted one by one, with material drawn from Seacole's own memoir, observations from the time (largely newspaper reports and war memoirs by officers) and later reference works. The ten myths are:

1. That Seacole won medals for bravery, variously numbered from one to four.

2. That, at the beginning of the war, she travelled to London to apply to be a nurse for ordinary soldiers and when she was rejected, went out to establish her own hospital.

3. That she frequently risked her life on the battlefield to save soldiers, on both sides, saving 'thousands.'

4. That her bankruptcy was the result of the sudden end of the war.

5. That, after the war, she volunteered to nurse in the Indian mutiny, but was again refused.

6. That she successfully treated such serious illnesses as cholera and yellow fever.

7. That she was a 'pioneer nurse,' the first 'nurse practitioner,' and gave her life's work to the early development of nursing.

8. That, unlike Nightingale, she was more than a nurse, but a doctor and pharmacist.

9. That she was black, a 'black nurse' and a 'black heroine.'

10. That Nightingale rejected her as a nurse for the Crimea, possibly for reasons of race, and continued to oppose her as late as the Franco-Prussian War in 1870.

All these myths appear in various combinations in many sources: printed books, articles and newspapers, the websites of major national institutions, television films, Youtube, school websites, Facebook and blogs. Print sources will normally be given first, for they often influenced the other media. For all of the myths, there are multiple sources, some normally considered to be reputable. To avoid repetition, examples have been kept to major misstatements, with (selected) reference to other errors.[1]

Myth 1: Medals, how many? Who awarded them?

That Seacole won medals is the oldest of the myths and the only one that clearly dates back to Seacole herself. Source after source credits her with having won from one to four medals for bravery: the (British) Crimea medal, the French Légion d'Honneur, the Turkish Medjidie and, some say, a medal from the Russians, while other sources mention the Sardinians. If she had won any of them, surely she would have described the award ceremony and all the happy details in her memoir. After all, she admitted on page 1 her love of 'the pomp, pride and circumstance of glorious war.' Having described attending the ceremony where the Order of the Bath was awarded to senior officers, she would hardly have neglected to relate a ceremony in which she was honoured. Winning any medal would have been remarkable at that time, for women were not then eligible for military medals.

A *Times* report in 1856 refers to her touring Crimean sites and disposing of her stock, with the curious mention that the sultan had sent her a medal, but that she was expecting to get one from the English government.[2] This shows that she *wanted* the Crimea medal, but did not receive it.

It seems that Seacole did not wear any medals while in the Crimea, although, according to her major biographer, Robinson, she may have acquired them there, by gift or purchase (167). Seacole's memoir makes no claim that she won any medals and her picture on the cover shows none.

---

[1] A website provides many further examples of misinformation, with documentation to the contrary: www.maryseacole.info/.

[2] From our special correspondent, 'The British Army,' *The Times* 16 May 1856 10C.

She was first seen wearing medals — no less than four — at her first bankruptcy court hearing, on 7 November 1856. Her purpose in wearing them was presumably to gain sympathy for her plight, and the coverage, in fact, was highly sympathetic to her.[3] She presumably did not wear the medals at the festival for her in July 1857, for that likely would have been noted in the extensive newspaper coverage of her appearances there.

The facts regarding the British Crimea medal are clear: the medal was for service, not requiring any particular act of bravery — the Victoria Cross was given 'for valour.' Clasps were added to the Crimea medal to indicate participation in particular battles (Alma, Balaclava and Inkermann); for the Sebastopol clasp, the recipient had to have been present at the siege from beginning to end. There was also an Azoff clasp for the navy, which similarly had a precise required period of service.[4]

No woman won the Crimea medal for the obvious reason that no woman was enlisted in the military. Nightingale was given a special brooch by Queen Victoria, inscribed 'Blessed are the Merciful' (2:500), presumably as the next best thing. The first awarding of medals to British women took place in 1883 with the Royal Red Cross; Nightingale, with various royal and noble women and a number of nurses from the Egyptian War, was on the first list of award winners (2:501).

War memoirs report award ceremonies for the Crimea medal. Major Astley, for example, described one held by Lord Rokeby on 20 September 1855, the anniversary of the Battle of the Alma. He joked on receiving his that he intended to wear it with his bed clothes. After the ceremony, they sat down to an 'Alma' dinner cooked by Soyer, for which he, Astley, furnished a sheep and ten brace of quail.[5]

The list of recipients of the Légion d'Honneur is kept by the Archives Nationales de France, available online for winners between 1803 and

---

[3] 'In re Seacole and Day,' *The Times* 7 November 1856 9B.

[4] John Horsley Mayo, *Medals and Decorations of the British Army and Navy* 2:374–75.

[5] Astley, *Fifty Years of my Life* 148–49.

1914. Seacole's name is not there. An inquiry to the Musée de la Légion d'Honneur in Paris elicited the information that they could find no trace of her being nominated.[6]

The Turkish Medjidie and French Légion d'Honneur were effectively also military medals, given to officers and men on nomination by the British Army. Commanding officers distributed them, as they did the Crimea medal. A letter home from another officer describes his receipt of the Medjidie.[7]

Robinson, while highly partial to her subject, did not buy the medals myth. She looked for mention of Seacole's name on award lists in the *London Gazette*, but found none. She suggested that it was 'more likely that Seacole "distinguished" herself' than that she had won any medals (167). Yet, even one of the better articles, in my view, credits her 'three medals awarded for her services to the military'[8] and repeats the error with a complaint that 'despite being decorated by the English, French and Turkish authorities, she was quickly erased from the public narrative of British imperial heroism' and was not given a statue with Sidney Herbert (202).

The frequent claim that Seacole was awarded the Medjidie medal is particularly curious, for she had no contact with Turkish soldiers. The Turkish commander, Omar Pasha, was an esteemed customer at her hut — although Muslim, he liked sherry and champagne (*WA* 110). She went out on horseback one day with him to observe a Turkish skirmish, but did not take food or drink for soldiers or give first aid. Moreover, her comments on Turks in general were derogatory: 'the degenerate descendants of the fierce Arabs' (106), 'deliberate, slow and indolent'

---

[6] Http://www.culture.gouv.fr/documentation/minitel. Email 4 September 2012 from the Musée de la Légion d'Honneur to Dr Gérard Vallée.

[7] William Allan, *Crimean Letters: From the 41st (the Welch) Regiment 1854–56* 150.

[8] Anita Rupprecht, '"Wonderful Adventures of Mrs Seacole in Many Lands" (1857): Colonial Identity and the Geographical Imagination' in David Lambert and Alan Lester, eds., *Colonial Lives Across the British Empire: Imperial Careering in the Long Nineteenth Century* 177.

who broke off 'into endless interruptions for the sacred duties of eating and praying, and getting into out-of-the-way corners at all times of the day to smoke themselves to sleep' (109).

By wearing the medals, Seacole was committing no offence. It only became a crime to wear medals not one's own in the UK Army Act of 1955, Section 197. The act has since been revised, but the same prohibition still holds. Specifically, the offence is to wear any military decoration, badge, stripe or emblem without authorization and to falsely represent oneself as being entitled to wear such. Exemptions have been made for widows and other family members of war veterans.

Statements perpetuating the myth that Seacole won medals are common and include institutions that ought to know better. The Guy's and St Thomas' NHS Foundation Trust, for example, was unambiguous: 'In acknowledgment of her courage and compassion during the war, she received four medals, including the Crimean Medal and the Légion d'Honneur.'[9] The website of the Mary Seacole Memorial Statue Appeal shows the medals and the description of the proposed statue states that the medals are to be prominent.[10] However, the designer selected, Martin Jennings, subsequently said that there would be no medals on the statue.[11] An Early Day Motion, supported by 179 MPs, regretted that the Crimean medal was the *only* recognition she got and urged government funding for a statue to give her more recognition.[12]

The Introduction to the first reissue of *Wonderful Adventures* adds verisimilitude by asserting that two of Seacole's medals are held at the Institute of Jamaica. It acknowledges that they cannot be 'verified from

---

[9] Karen Sorenson, 'Mary Seacole Memorial Statue Update,' Guy's and St Thomas' NHS Foundation Trust 20 July 2011.

[10] Mary Seacole Memorial Statue Appeal, 7 July 2012.

[11] Jennings email to author 29 October 2012; his email of 17 January 2014 states that no medals are shown on the statue maquette.

[12] Early Day Motion 744, introduced by Roy Beggs 11 March 2004.

official sources,'[13] omitting the salient fact that the Institute has no record of how the medals got there or whose they were. Repeated inquiries elicited the information that it owns two medals, the French Legion of Honour and the Turkish Medjidie, but possesses no documentation connecting them with Seacole or explaining how and when they were added to the collection.[14]

Hugh Small, in falling for the medal myth, called it 'an extraordinary departure from the rules,' which it would have been had it happened. He also made a point of saying that Nightingale was *not* awarded the medal, despite Lord Palmerston's efforts to get one for her.[15]

A biographical source of the National Library of Jamaica has Seacole 'presented with the Crimean medal, which she always wore afterwards on her dress.'[16] The website of 100 Black Britons claims that 'she was awarded a Crimean medal.'[17] The Seacole entry in the *Oxford Dictionary of National Biography* is more circumspect: it does not state that she won medals, but shows a picture of the Gleichen bust, where she wore four, without noting that they were not hers.[18] The National Portrait Gallery's website 'Focus on Seacole' similarly, short of expressly stating that she won any, repeatedly shows her wearing medals, without clarifying that she had not won them. The medals myth appears in an editorial[19] and two

---

[13] Ziggi Alexander and Audrey Dewjee, eds, *Wonderful Adventures of Mrs Seacole* 36.

[14] Email from Dr Jonathan Greenland, Institute of Jamaica 10 December 2012.

[15] Hugh Small, *Avenging Angel* 200.

[16] 'Mary Seacole (1805–1881),' *Biographies of Jamaican Personalities*. Online www.nlu.gov.jm/bios-p-z).

[17] 'Mary Seacole. Crimean War Veteran Nurse and Original Lady of the Lamp,' online 2005.

[18] Alan Palmer, 'Seacole née Grant, Mary Jane, 1805–1881,' *Oxford Dictionary of National Biography*.

[19] 'Seacole Portrait Takes Rightful Place,' *Nursing Standard* 19,18 (12 January 2005):4.

articles in the *Nursing Standard*, the first of which states that the Russians also gave her a medallion,[20] a point to be addressed under Myth 3. Even a major medical history of the Crimean War has Seacole with one medal, the Crimean.[21] Anionwu vigorously defended the medals claim as late as 2013, in an article which also claims Seacole to be a 'social reformer,' along with Nightingale and Elizabeth Fry. Her arguments, however, repeat the fact of medals being held at the Institute of Jamaica and their being mentioned in an obituary of her sister as evidence that they were awarded her, although neither source gave any evidence of where the medals came from.[22] That Seacole wore them in photographs, a portrait and a bust does not clear up the mystery of who originally won them.

A *Guardian* online contribution has Seacole being 'awarded several medals for bravery.' This item also incorrectly states that she set up the 'British Hotel' in Turkey (in fact, a hut-store in the Crimea) and gave 'food and care to British soldiers close to battle lines.'[23] Another electronic source, which calls Seacole a 'dignified Afro-Caribbean,' has her awarded three medals, with all the usual stories of the heroism she displayed nursing on the battlefield. It also says that she provided the men, at her own expense, 'a mess table of home cooking, comfort, convalescence and food for their spirit' and later has her meeting 'the royal family.'[24] But her mess table was for officers, not soldiers, as her memoir made abundantly clear, and there is no evidence that she ever met the royal family. A story in *The Independent* in 2010 says Seacole was

---

[20] 'Elizabeth Anionwu Discovers Mary Seacole was a Celebrity in her Time,' *Nursing Standard* 24,5 (7 October 2009):26; Sidone Chifulya, 'Inspiring Stories,' *Nursing Standard* 25,5 (6 October 2010):72.

[21] Shepherd, *Crimean Doctors* 507.

[22] Elizabeth Anionwu, 'Scotching Three Myths About Mary Seacole,' *British Journal of Healthcare Assistants* 7,10 (October 2013):309–11.

[23] Tim Campbell, 'A Hero of the Crimean War,' *The Guardian* 12 October 2008.

[24] Athena Krambides, 'Finding Mary Seacole in London,' *Culture* 24, 11 December 2006.

awarded 'four medals including the Crimean Medal and the Légion d'Honneur, in recognition of her courage.'[25]

A biographical note on Seacole in a reissue of a war journal by an officer's wife, *Mrs Duberly's War*, credits her with being 'a familiar sight at the front tending the wounding, and after the war was awarded the Crimean medal.'[26] Seacole, however, could hardly have been a familiar sight at the front, since she was present at only three battles and entirely missed the three major ones. Mrs Duberly did not mention Seacole at all in her original 1856 publication.[27]

The hour-long Channel 4 film 'Mary Seacole: The Real Angel of the Crimea,' 2005, makes the claim that Seacole won four medals. The thirty-minute BBC educational film also has her 'honoured with four medals,' 'for bravery, kindness and saving lives.' It further states that two of the medals were preserved in Jamaica but, as noted above, the Institute of Jamaica has no documentation to indicate their provenance. That 'educational' film also shows the Gleichen bust, without qualification, with four medals.

The BBC's Famous People website has Seacole winning medals from Britain, Turkey and France for her 'bravery,' with a picture of a Crimea medal with four clasps — presumably the medal she won, although it does not say that. Quite apart from the fact that the Crimea medal was given only to the military, it was awarded for service, not bravery, requiring presence at particular battles. 'Famous People' is part of the BBC's Schools Series.

The electronic *Caribbean History Archives* adds new twists and turns to the medals myth, claiming not only that Seacole won three, but that the queen herself decorated her 'on more than one occasion.' But then Seacole was, according to that source, well known to the royal family and

---

[25] Chris Green, 'Memorial to Crimea's black nurse in danger,' *The Independent* 25 January 2010.

[26] Christine Kelly, note, in Frances Isabella Duberly, *Mrs Duberly's War: Journal and Letters from the Crimea 1854–6* 323.

[27] Mrs Henry Duberly, *Journal Kept During the Russian War from the Departure of the Army from England in April 1854 to the Fall of Sebastopol.*

a frequent guest for tea at Buckingham Palace. A fake dialogue is provided with Seacole descending from her carriage, although she did not own one or use one, telling the guardsmen that 'the royal family is glad any time to ask me to tea.'[28]

Children's books also convey the medals myth with pictures of Seacole wearing them, without any explanation that they were not hers.[29] One such book claims the British Crimea medal, the French Légion d'Honneur and the Turkish Medjidie for her.[30] Another turns her business, in practice called 'Mrs Seacole's store' or 'Mrs Seacole's hut,' into a 'boarding house, canteen and a general store' popular with the troops, when in fact it was for officers.[31] That book also has Seacole meeting the royal family after the Crimean War (18), when, in fact, Nightingale did this, not Seacole. A Channel 4 children's book has a picture of the two medals Seacole is supposed to have won;[32] it errs also in portraying her on the cover as a nurse in a blue uniform with a white apron and cap.

Seacole contributed enormously to the medals myth by being painted, sculpted and photographed wearing them. While the first bust of her, done in 1859, has no medals, the 1869 oil painting by Albert Charles Challen features three. The person who found the portrait and later sold it to the National Gallery explained that 'none of the medals' on the portrait could be 'conclusively identified' and that the ribbons were wrong for the medals.[33] Gleichen's 1871 bust shows her 'adorned with her Crimean

---

[28] Gerard A. Bresson, 'Mary Seacole,' *Caribbean History Archives*, accessed 28 February 2012.

[29] For example, Emma Lynch, *The Life of Mary Seacole* 6, 22 and 24.

[30] Eric L Huntley, *Two Lives: Florence Nightingale and Mary Seacole.*

[31] Paul Harrison, *Who Was Mary Seacole?* 14.

[32] Christine Moorcroft and Magnus Magnusson, *Mary Seacole 1805–1881* 19.

[33] Rappaport, reply to Glenn A. Christodoulou, 'Honouring Seacole,' *History Today* March 2005 online.

medals,' four of them.[34] Robinson suggested that he might have loaned them for the sitting (214). Or (my guess) he might have loaned her the Medjidie, which does not appear in any other picture or bust of her. That bust was copied by George Kelly, again with four medals. It is used on the website of Science Museum: Exploring the History of Medicine, again without any explanation that they were not hers.

Three medals appear in the black and white photograph Seacole commissioned for a carte de visite in 1873. An undated black and white photograph, discovered at Winchester College, has her wearing four ribbons.[35]

Queen Elizabeth II was drawn into the medals hoax when she opened the Mary Seacole Building at Brunel University. She made no comments herself, but is pictured beside a Seacole plaque which reproduces the Challen portrait (with three medals) and gives an unusually fallacious statement of what Seacole did to earn them.[36]

Myth 2: Travelling to London to apply to become a nurse to care for ordinary soldiers, then going to the Crimea to establish her own hospital when she was refused

The real story of how Seacole decided she wanted to go to the Crimea to nurse, set out in Chapter 3, lacks the right stuff for the Seacole myth. Many sources give the new, improved version: that she went to London from Jamaica deliberately to apply to become an army nurse. In fact she went to London to deal with her gold mining stocks and, only after spending some time trying to realize a profit, to no avail, did she decide to go to the war (74).

---

[34] 'Sculpture in the Studio,' *The Times* 21 July 1871 4E.

[35] 'Mary Seacole's Signature Found,' *The Gleaner* 26 June 2009.

[36] 19 May 2006 opening of Mary Seacole Building, Brunel University.

A *Times* story in 1954, on the centenary of the start of the Crimean War, paints Seacole, when refused as a nurse, as 'undaunted' and determined to find another way to bring help 'to her beloved lads in the Army and Navy.' She and her partner were then said to have raised funds (when, in fact, they used their profits from previous enterprises) 'to start a canteen at the seat of the war,' when their real object was a mess table for officers. The story creates a glorified perception of egalitarian relations between officers and ordinary soldiers, melding the canteen for soldiers with the mess table for officers, inventing a place 'where officers and men could come and taste her expert cooking of English and West Indian dishes.'[37]

The above-noted entry on Seacole in the *Oxford Companion to Black British History* has fewer errors than most sources, but even it perpetuates misinformation on her sailing to London to apply to nurse in the Crimean War, 'expecting a grateful welcome,' when her own memoir is clear that her purpose in going to London was to attend to her gold stocks (74).

To make Seacole's trip to the Crimea even more heroic, some commentators suggest that she made the voyage alone. An entry in *Who's Who in British History,* for example, states that Seacole, 'undeterred' by being turned down, made 'the nearly 4,000-mile journey to the Crimea alone.'[38] But this is unlikely, given that the same two black servants, Mac and Mary, who were with her in Panama (*WA* 12, 36, 39, 57–58), turn up also in the Crimea (113). The Unison Campaign similarly has Seacole making 'the 4,000 mile journey by herself.'[39] The BBC, in its Learning Zone series, has Seacole travelling 'alone to nurse soldiers on the battlefield,' along with numerous other errors.[40]

---

[37] 'Mrs Seacole: A West Indian Nurse in the Crimea,' *The Times* 24 December 1954 8E.

[38] Juliet Gardiner, ed., 'Seacole, Mary,' *Who's Who in British History*.

[39] Unison, 'The Mary Seacole (1805–1880) Campaign "Turn her into Stone,"' 16/1/10.

[40] BBC Learning Zone, 'The Work of Florence Nightingale and Mary Seacole' (drama). Classic Clips 5.44 clip 13650, first broadcast March 2012.

Some commentators also attest that Seacole, when she was not accepted by the War Office as a hospital nurse, opened and managed her own hospital, battlefield hospital or clinic. Conservative minister for public health, Anne Milton, called Seacole's hut 'a makeshift hospital where she saved lives on a daily basis.'[41] Historian John Peck called it not just a mess hall for officers, store and canteen, but a 'medical dispensary and sick bay.'[42] Historian Trevor Royle called Seacole's establishment a 'rough and ready nursing station,'[43] all the more remarkable an achievement because Nightingale had 'rejected her offer' to nurse (257). Stevenhoved called it a 'free casualty ward at the hotel.'[44] Rappaport's Seacole entry in her *Encyclopedia of Women Social Reformers* has her running a 'sick bay where she nursed the wounded, dispensed her own herbal medicines and introduced methods of nursing that emphasized cleanliness, plenty of ventilation and an abundance of her own home-cooked food' (2:631). However, Seacole's own memoir never mentions a sick bay. It gives no specifics about the canteen, except that it was for 'the soldiery' (114). The dispensing took place while she cooked meals for officers (140); her memoir also made clear that the home-cooked food (by her and her two cooks) was for sale to officers, not the men. She never discussed ventilation or cleanliness in regards to her hut — nor are huts known for their ventilation. Soyer's memoir corroborates the food and drink focus of the operation, with further details about the social side (see Chapter 3, p 74–75).

A Dutch journal article, based on a dissertation, repeats the usual mistakes about Seacole going to offer her services, being denied and then establishing, at her own expense, 'a British hotel where she tended the wounded soldiers,' offering them not only 'bandages and medicines, but

---

[41] 'An Inspiration: The Mary Seacole Awards,' *Community Practitioner* 84,12 (December 2011):4.

[42] John Peck, *War, the Army and Victorian Literature* 36.

[43] Trevor Royle, *Crimea: The Great Crimean War 1854–1856* 256.

[44] Susanne Stevenhoved, 'Mary Grant Seacole,' *Six Hundred Women and One Man: Nurses on Stamps* 33.

also refreshments, wine and lemonade.'[45] According to an American nursing textbook, Seacole's hut had a 'top floor arranged like a hospital,' where she nursed sick soldiers. It also had her serving as a nurse in Cuba and Panama 'during the yellow fever and cholera epidemics' and even conducting 'forensic studies.'[46]

Commentators at the time did not use the advertised name, the 'British Hotel,' but the more homely 'Mrs Seacole's hut' or simply 'Mrs Seacole's.' Her friend Soyer refers to it as 'the Seacole tavern.'[47] A Soyer biographer calls it an 'unofficial canteen' and a 'tin hut.'[48] A newspaper story refers to her 'iron storehouse with wooden sheds.'[49] Lady Alicia Blackwood calls it an 'omnibus shop.'[50] An officer's memoir calls it 'a sort of eating house.'[51] Dr Buzzard's description is 'a store...where, in an emergency, one could obtain some kind of a meal.'[52] A *Times* item after the war calls it a 'provision store.'[53] A book on Raglan mentions it as a 'tolerable restaurant in Kadikoi' calling Seacole herself a 'kind-hearted Jamaican mulatto.'[54]

---

[45] Marijke Huisman, 'Autobiography and Contemporary History: The Dutch Reception of Autobiographies, 1850–1918,' accessed 15 December 2013, a translation of 'Beter dan Thucydides en Wagenaar...Autobiografieen en de geshiedenis van de eigen tijd, 1850–1918,' *Tijdschrift voor Geschiedenis* 118,4 (2005):513.

[46] Barbara Cherry and Susan R. Jacob, 'Mary Seacole,' in *Contemporary Nursing: Issues, Trends and Management* 9.

[47] Soyer, *Culinary Campaign* 479.

[48] Morris, *Portrait of a Chef* 165.

[49] 'The Fall of Sebastopol,' *The Times* 26 September 1855 8A.

[50] Blackwood, *Narrative of Personal Experiences* 262.

[51] Astley, *Fifty Years of My Life* 145.

[52] Buzzard, *With the Turkish Army in the Crimea* 179.

[53] 'Mrs Seacole,' *The Times* 5 July 1856 10C.

[54] Hibbert, *The Destruction of Lord Raglan* 260.

Some ten years after the war, a British visitor to the Crimea remarked on what was left 'of Mrs Seacole's famous store': an 'immense heap of broken bottles by the roadside, glittering in the sunlight, like thousands of black diamonds.'[55]

One nursing textbook states that Seacole, after being refused even an interview because of 'her race and ethnicity,' went to the Crimea where 'she soon established a hospital and respite home for wounded and fatigued soldiers.'[56] Another has Seacole, after being refused by Nightingale, borrowing money to get to the war zone, where 'she set up a private hotel for British soldiers.'[57] A story in the American magazine *The New Yorker* says Seacole constructed 'a hotel-clinic from scrap where she handed out wine and hot tea to the soldiers,' who, of course, 'loved her.'[58] Her memoir never mentions giving out wine or tea to soldiers at her hut, which was never a hotel-clinic.

In a book chapter with a literary focus, Seacole is described as a 'voluntary member of the British military machine,' whose 'aptly named "British Hotel" offered British soldiers reasonably priced food, a comfortable meeting place and Seacole's expert medical care.' She 'supplied British soldiers with meat, tea, coffee, linens, medicines, fruit, wine and doctoring at the British Hotel.'[59] Yet the food was available only to officers and was expensive even for them.

Simon Schama's description of Seacole's hut in his *History of Britain* is one of the most far-fetched: 'a combination of supply depot, refectory for soldiers about to go into action, and nursing and recovery station for the

---

[55] Robert Arthur Arnold, *From the Levant, the Black Sea and the Danube* 2:184.

[56] Marilyn Klainberg, *An Historical Overview of Nursing* 26.

[57] Margaret McAllister and John B. Lowe, *The Resilient Nurse: Empowering Your Practice* 26.

[58] Ian Frazier, 'Two Nurses,' *The New Yorker* 25 April 2011.

[59] Deirdre H. McMahon, '"My Own Dear Sons": Discursive Maternity and Proper British Bodies in *Wonderful Adventures of Mrs Seacole in Many Lands*,' 183 and 188.

sick and wounded' (3:220). He compared it favourably with Nightingale's hospital, being 'unlike the Scutari wards...warm and dry' (3:220–21). No doubt the hut where Seacole served officers champagne was warm and dry, but there was no nursing or recovery station in it at all, warm or cold, dry or wet. He was right in referring to the 'deathtrap' hospital at Scutari (3:221), but the conditions there were the result of gross defects in toilets, drains and sewers that were overlooked in the army's inspection.

A Jamaica commemorative stamp in 1991, labeled 'Mary Seacole Nursing in Hospital in Scutari,' shows her in a nurse's uniform at the bedside of a soldier. A reference book on stamps, however, gives an unequivocal explanation that 'she did not participate in the care of any of the wounded soldiers in Scutari, as portrayed on the Jamaican stamp issued in 1991.'[60]

A children's book brings together several inaccuracies. It claims that while Nightingale was the 'better known' nurse, she was not the only one 'capable of organizing hospitals in the Crimea.' The other, a 'respected nurse,' was 'all but ignored,' turned down because of her race. She then set up a hospital 'near the battlefields' and 'many nurses' worked with her.[61] Seacole, it says, 'was on the scene to help treat and care for the soldiers as they were injured, or fell ill, saving many lives' (25). But Seacole never described any hospital as hers and none of her employees were nurses; she employed cooks and animal handlers, plus her maid. She never mentioned soldiers suddenly falling ill on the battlefield and this is difficult to imagine, for battles were short: the three Seacole witnessed were over in a few hours.

The website for 100 Black Britons calls Seacole a 'Veteran Nurse and Original Lady of the Lamp,' presumably a dig at Nightingale. Seacole, however, is not known to have carried a lamp through hospital wards, for she was not on night duty at any time she was in a hospital, which she attended only as a visitor. An Early Day Motion, signed by 179 MPs of

---

[60] Stevenhoved, *Six Hundred Women* 33.

[61] Kay Barnham, *Florence Nightingale: The Lady of the Lamp* 24.

all parties, echoed the 'original "lady with the lamp"' claim.[62] The BBC repeated it, with numerous other misstatements, in its coverage of the Black Britons award.[63]

Myth 3: Heroism on the battlefield, risking her life for ordinary soldiers, on both sides

Apart from the medals myth, there are many associated statements that claim Seacole was a heroine on the battlefield. She acknowledged in her memoir, before leaving for the war, her *desire* to become a 'Crimean heroine' (76), but made no claim of actual heroism in the book. Such claims are quite recent. An article on Seacole as 'the first nurse practitioner' has her, among many other errors and exaggerations, helping wounded soldiers on the battlefields 'even while the battles were still raging.'[64]

Rappaport's *Encyclopedia* entry has Seacole 'riding out alone on her mule with supplies of food and drink and medicine for the wounded' (2:632), although she herself described the battlefield excursions as being on horseback, with an employee to handle the two mules, which were laden with supplies of food and drink for officers and spectators. She also gave food and drink to those who could not pay, presumably soldiers, and described doing first aid work, bandaging and sewing up wounds on the spot. Her memoir shows her to have been generous, as do other accounts, but, fundamentally, Seacole was running a business, with the pro bono work on the side, and made this quite clear. On her last excursion with mules, to the fallen Sebastopol, she went with her business partner and many friends and described it as a social occasion (173).

---

[62] Sponsored by Roy Beggs, 2 March 2004.

[63] BBC One Minute World News 10 February 2004.

[64] P.R. Messmer and Y. Parchment, 'Mary Grant Seacole: The First Nurse Practitioner,' *Clinical Excellence for Nurse Practitioners* 2,1 (February 1998):47.

Some of the claims of heroism are ludicrous, such as Seacole actually nursing the *sick* on the battlefield. For this to have happened, army doctors and orderlies must have moved patients out of their hospitals onto the battlefield, hoping that she would come by. Yet the Seacole Memorial Statue Appeal paints a picture of her riding out 'to the front line' with 'baskets of medicines of her own preparation to treat the sick and wounded of both sides on the battlefields.'[65] The Russians, too, it would have us believe, moved their sick onto the battlefield in order to get her help! Nor is there any evidence that Seacole personally prepared the 'baskets of medicines,' which, in her memoir, she said she purchased in London (81–82).

A nursing journal editorial refers to Seacole tending 'the sick and wounded' at the front, 'with her medical bag on one mule and hams and wine on another,'[66] an embellishment of her own account. The dean of Health Sciences and Social Care at Brunel University also claimed that Seacole provided 'health care and nursing for the sick and injured on the battlefield.'[67] The BBC History website has her, not only nursing the sick and wounded, but giving everyone food, blankets, clean clothes and kindness, even 'when battles were raging.' Nightingale did provide blankets, clean clothes, etc., but not while battles were raging.

A children's book credits Seacole with having 'searched the battlefields for wounded and dying men, even while the guns were still firing,' which would have been heroic indeed, if it had happened. She was later visited by soldiers, it said, 'whose lives she had saved,' visits which do not appear in her memoir or anyone else's.[68] She also became 'as familiar a face in military hospitals as she was in the thick

---

[65] Mary Seacole Memorial Statue Appeal website 7 July 2012.

[66] James P. Smith, 'Mary Jane Seacole 1805–1881: A Black British Nurse,' *Journal of Advanced Nursing* 9,5 (1984):427.

[67] Lorraine H. De Souza, speech at opening of Mary Seacole building 19 May 2006.

[68] Castor, *Mary Seacole* 34.

of battle tending the wounded where they lay.'[69] For none of this is there any evidence.

The myth that Seacole treated men on 'both sides' is a popular feature in Seacole lore, often, it is claimed, while 'under fire.' It appears in the *Nursing Standard*, the journal of the Royal College of Nursing.[70] The nursing union Unison used it in its statement of support for a Seacole statue.[71] The Nottingham University Hospitals NHS Trust repeated the claim when naming its stroke ward after Seacole.[72] The BBC's half hour Knowledge film has her not only helping 'soldiers on both sides,' but being herself injured in battle.[73]

The claim that Seacole helped 'both sides' appears in teaching materials, for example, in a website giving advice for preparing for the GCSE History examination. A preferred answer to the question, 'What points determine the difference between Mary Seacole and Florence Nightingale?' is: 'Seacole often tended wounded from both sides actually on the battlefield and under fire,' which Nightingale never did. The answer also disputes Nightingale as the founder of modern nursing, holding that the two were 'equally important in improving medical care and treatment of injured soldiers.'[74]

The 'both sides' theme appears on a website of a Government of Trinidad institute,[75] an online newspaper story[76] and descriptions of

---

[69] Graeme Donald, *Loose Cannons: 101 Myths, Mishaps and Misadventures of Military History* 66.

[70] Sidone Chifulya, 'Inspiring Stories,' *Nursing Standard* 25,5 (6 October 2010):72.

[71] 'The Mary Seacole (1805–1880) Campaign "Turn her into Stone"' 16/1/10.

[72] *Nottingham Post* news release 8 October 2009.

[73] BBC Knowledge, 'Mary Seacole: A Hidden History.'

[74] Online for GCSE History, posted 14 June 2011.

[75] National Institute of Higher Education, Research, Science and Technology, 'A Caribbean Florence Nightingale: Mary Seacole, Nurse.'

Seacole stamps.[77] The Wikipedia entry also made the claim, although the point was subsequently dropped.

Seacole's own claim of treating wounded Russians is confined to one battle, the Tchernaya, where she said she attended to several only. One unfortunate Russian bit her as she tried to remove a bullet from his mouth; another gave her a ring in thanks for the 'little use' she was to him (166). Also pertinent, but not mentioned, is that, after that same battle, she helped herself to a Russian metal cross and cut souvenir buttons off the coats of dead Russian soldiers. After the Russians left Sebastopol, a French soldier sold her a painting of a Madonna stolen from a church (176). She was given a decorated altar candle, also stolen from a Sebastopol church, which she subsequently gave to the duke of Cambridge, later commander-in-chief of the British Army, at the end of the war (174). None of the sources cited above acknowledged Seacole's looting or her acceptance of loot from soldiers.

The 'saving thousands' claim appears in the BBC's advertising for its 2000 film, 'Mary Seacole: A Hidden History.' The *Nursing Standard* echoed the advertisement when the film was rebroadcast, stating also that Seacole was rejected by Nightingale's organization but 'got to the front line at her own expense and risk' where 'she saved thousands of British soldiers.'[78] Designating the number of lives saved as 'thousands' is recent, and far from any claim Seacole, or her most enthusiastic supporters during or following the war, ever made.

A history website opens with the declaration that Seacole 'fought colour prejudice to save lives on the battlefield and earn the love of thousands.' Army 'medics,' it says, were 'lost in admiration' for her, although it named not one. Seacole 'was more accomplished, more courageous and just as dedicated' as Nightingale, the website asserts,

---

[76] Kevin O'Brien Chang, 'Black Woman Pioneer Mary Seacole,' *The Gleaner* 26 July 2012.

[77] Stevenhoved, *Six Hundred Women* 33.

[78] 'Pick of the Week,' *Nursing Standard* 19,25 (2 March 2005):28.

but was forgotten because of her skin colour. In Jamaica, she had become 'probably the world's leading authority on cholera.'[79]

The website of the Mary Seacole House in Liverpool credits her with saving 'thousands of men' from 'cholera, dysentery and jaundice' thanks to her 'ample medical knowledge and skills...and...caring bedside manner.' Yet we now know her medical 'knowledge' included recourse to toxic substances.[80]

Myth 4: Bankruptcy caused by the sudden end of the war

According to currently circulating myths, supported by many sources, Seacole's bankruptcy was the result of circumstances beyond her control, in particular the sudden end of the Crimean War. This claim engenders sympathy for Seacole, for she did indeed suffer bankruptcy. In her memoir, however, she explains only that the war was ruinous for her (*WA* 189), without suggesting suddenness.

Rappaport's *Encyclopedia* story, already cited for other errors, is an example here of the 'sudden end' claim (2:632). As explained in Chapter 2, there was a long gap from the last battle, on 8 September 1855, and the peace treaty signed on 30 March 1856. Business was booming at Mrs Seacole's all the while: 'My restaurant was always full,' she noted in her memoir (178). And, as proprietors of successful businesses are wont to do, she and her partner made 'extensive additions to our store and out houses — our shelves were filled with articles laid in at a great cost' (189).

The National Portrait Gallery also makes the false claim that the 'sudden end of the war' left her bankrupt.[81] A variation on the victim theme can be

---

[79] Brian Baker, 'The Forgotten War Nurse who Outshone Florence Nightingale,' UK/Irish History suite 101, 17 August 2011.

[80] The day centre opened in 1999, but when the 'thousands' claim appeared on the website is not apparent.

[81] National Portrait Gallery online, 'Lost Portrait of Mary Seacole Discovered' 10 January 2005.

seen in *The Times* story of 1954, where her bankruptcy is blamed on 'plundering' and 'pilfering' by people of many nations,[82] a claim contrary both to Seacole's memoir and her business partner's account of their losses.[83] The Science Museum's website attributes Seacole's bankruptcy to debts 'run up by soldiers,' although the debts of officers were only a negligible factor and soldiers were not given loans at all. The entry in an encyclopedia of African American women writers cites the 'sudden end' of the war, along with 'pilfering and disregarded IOUs' as causes of the bankruptcy.[84]

A book chapter blames Seacole's financial ruin after the 'sudden end' to the war to her destroying stock 'rather than trade with Russians.'[85] Her own memoir, however, suggests no objection to Russians, but only to the prices they would pay (*WA* 196).

Myth 5: Volunteering for the Indian Mutiny

Several authors state that Seacole offered to go to nurse in the Indian Mutiny in 1857, the year after the Crimean War ended. An article in a peer-reviewed medical journal claims that Seacole, when news of the Indian Mutiny reached Britain, was 'determined to go and provide a similar service to that which she had provided in the Crimea.'[86] The author quotes

---

[82] 'Mrs Seacole: A West Indian Nurse in the Crimea,' *The Times* 24 December 1954 8E.

[83] 'Mrs Seacole's Late Partner in the Crimea,' *The Times* 14 April 1857 7F.

[84] Natalie Morton, 'Mary Seacole (1805–1881),' in Yolanda Williams Page, ed., *Encyclopedia of African American Women Writers* 508.

[85] Deirdre H. McMahon, '"My Own Dear Sons": Discursive Maternity and Proper British Bodies in *Wonderful Adventures of Mrs Seacole in Many Lands*,' 183.

[86] Christine Short, 'Mary Seacole: Forgotten Hero?' *Scottish Medical Journal* 56,2 (May 2011):110–14. For a detailed refutation to this article, see Lynn McDonald, 'Florence Nightingtale and Mary Seacole: Which is the Forgotten Hero of Health Care and Why,' *Scottish Medical Journal* 59,1 (1 February 2014)"66–69.

no source and the only documentation available is indirect. Anthony Trollope's comment that Queen Victoria would not let her go because her life was 'too precious' has been noted in Chapter 3. A letter to the editor of the *Daily News*, by an anonymous Nightingale nurse in the Crimean War, announced her own willingness to go, with 'forty ladies,' with Seacole.[87] The letter writer identified herself only as having nursed five months at Scutari. This time period suggests the letter writer was likely either Elizabeth Blake or Margaret Williams,[88] both of whom were invalided home. The letter writer outlined her intent which was for the India volunteers to direct soldiers' wives as nurses, which the writer said had been done successfully at Scutari. This makes no sense, for Nightingale vehemently opposed the use of untrained women, especially soldiers' wives. That she would assign them to attend 'cases of extreme danger,' as the letter writer stated, is not credible. The letter got a reply from the East India Company, which was also published in the *Daily News*. It explained that no nurses were needed, as every station and force in the field had its own hospital, and that 'no European women would be allowed to follow the camp.'[89] A number of other newspapers picked up the story.

Seacole's hypothetical offer to nurse in India appears also in the online *Oxford Companion to Black British History*, which claims that 'she unsuccessfully volunteered to nurse victims of the Indian Mutiny in 1857,' mentioning also the Franco-Prussian War in 1870. No source is provided for either claim. As noted in Chapter 3, there is no evidence in the records of the war secretary, Lord Panmure, of any such offer for India. Nor does the timing work:

* The sepoys' objection to handling pig grease in preparing cartridges, contrary to Hindu practice, emerged in February 1857;
* The first violence broke out in March 1857;

---

[87] 'Letter from A Nurse in the late War,' *Daily News* 21 September 1857.

[88] Details in Wellcome Trust Ms 8995/78, *CW* 290.

[89] James C. Melvill letter, *Daily News* 21 September 1857.

* The first murders of British civilians took place in May 1857;

* In late May, Seacole indicated an interest in serving the British cause in China, or some other part of the empire, not mentioning India;

* On 18 July 1857, the above-noted former Nightingale nurse wrote the East India Company, mentioning 'ladies' going with Seacole to nurse in the mutiny, but the company's reply of 22 August stated that no women were wanted;

* On 1 October 1857, Seacole wrote the military secretary at the War Office to ask him to review an enclosed letter for the war secretary. However, the subject of said letter is unknown as the letter itself is missing and the covering letter does not state it. The reply, if the letter were about going to India, would likely have been the same as that by the East India Company, that no women nurses were wanted.

The one conflict where nurses would soon be needed was the American Civil War. By that time, 1861, Seacole was in nearby Jamaica, yet there is no suggestion that she ever considered going. Yet the need was desperate. Nurses were actively recruited and given brief hospital training.

One might also note the incongruity of Seacole's apparent willingness to go to China, or to a British colony somewhere, with her lack of interest in serving in a closer conflict, the American Civil War, where nurses were wanted.

Myths of nursing, medical practice and cures

For the next myths, on Seacole's reputed medical and nursing skills and cures, the material includes her time in Jamaica and Panama as well as during the Crimean War.

Myth 6: Successful cures for cholera and yellow fever

Seacole herself claimed very few cures for cholera and none for yellow fever. She openly acknowledged failures and blunders and regretted her inability to cure many people who came to her. One author, however, has her developing a medicine which 'cured yellow fever and cholera,'[90] although he did not name the medicine or its ingredients. An article on Seacole as 'the first nurse practitioner' has her nursing 'British soldiers during epidemics of cholera, dysentery and yellow fever in Jamaica, Cuba and Panama,'[91] although none of Seacole's (modest) claims for success concern Cuba, or dysentery as an epidemic — nor were British soldiers stationed in Panama or Cuba, for that matter. The website *Caribbean History Archives* credits both Seacole and her mother with being successful in curing yellow fever.[92]

A nursing book falsely states that Seacole 'expanded her nursing skills by travelling through the British colonies,' where she encountered and managed 'several epidemics of cholera and yellow fever.'[93] But Seacole's travels were all for business purposes: buying and selling things, bringing in supplies for her brother's hotel in Panama and then establishing her own restaurant/store. She dealt with epidemics if and when they occurred and never claimed to have 'managed' any of them. The yellow fever epidemic was at home in Jamaica and she acknowledged defeat (59–63).

Another nursing book, after incorrectly crediting her mother with teaching her nursing skills, has Seacole traveling 'as a nurse' to Cuba and Panama to work in cholera and yellow fever epidemics.[94] But her memoir mentions no epidemic when she visited Cuba (5) and her trip to Panama was for business. A serious, recent history of the Crimean War credits the 'extraordinary' woman with having 'worked as a nurse in the British military stations in Jamaica,'[95] which she herself never claimed.

---

[90] Huntley, *Two Lives: Florence Nightingale and Mary Seacole* 43.

[91] P.R. Messmer and Y. Parchment, 'Mary Grant Seacole: The First Nurse Practitioner,' *Clinical Excellence for Nurse Practitioners* 2,1 (February 1998):47.

[92] Gerard A. Bresson, 'Mary Seacole,' *Caribbean History Archives* 28 February 2012.

[93] McAllister and Lowe, *The Resilient Nurse* 25.

[94] Klainberg, *Historical Overview of Nursing* 26.

[95] Figes, *Crimea: The Last Crusade* 354.

In the yellow fever epidemic of 1853, Seacole recounted doing little apart from giving comfort to the dying. She was asked to take nurses to an army camp near Kingston, 'but it was little we could do to mitigate the severity of the epidemic' (63). On treating cholera, she frankly recorded having made 'no doubt...some lamentable blunders' and might have 'lost patients which a little later I could have saved.' Notes on the cholera medicines she found later made her 'shudder' (31). Given that she used mercury and lead, she had reason to.

Schama's *History of Britain* describes Seacole as having 'acquired a reputation for working miracles of recuperation among the critically sick':

> Her antidotes for dysenteric diseases and the associated dehydration which almost always proved fatal were all drawn from the Caribbean botanical pharmacopeia. This origin guaranteed that they would be ridiculed as 'barbarous' potions by the medical establishment and that Mary's application to go to the Crimea to treat the cholera and typhoid victims (which accounted for the vast majority of fatalities) would be dismissed out of hand, not least by Nightingale herself (3:220).

However, we do not know what was in that 'Caribbean botanical pharmacopeia,' or even how Caribbean it was, since she purchased her Crimea supplies in London and had not been in the Caribbean for some time. Mercury chloride and lead acetate are hardly part of the 'botanical pharmacopeia.' Schama misleads also in his reference to her countering dehydration, for Seacole's remedies would have intensified it: emetics, sweating and purging through the bowels. The effective treatment in use now (with death rates under 1%) is oral rehydration therapy, a far cry from the metallic pharmacopeia utilized by Seacole and many doctors. Schama errs also in supposing that the medical establishment would have rejected her remedies — for they were very much in line with medical opinion of the day.

In her memoir, Seacole described giving first aid on a few occasions and other people who saw her gave her credit for timely help. She was generous in providing tea, lemonade and cake to soldiers at the wharf — before her huts were ready for business — but made no claim to have saved lives by this or pioneered treatments.

Myth 7: That Seacole was a 'pioneer nurse,' the first 'nurse practitioner' and gave her 'life's work' to develop nursing

The projected Seacole statue at St Thomas' is to identify Seacole as 'Pioneer Nurse,' at Nightingale's hospital no less. Supporters use the term 'nurse' for Seacole as if it were a fact, although she never called herself one, never took anything akin to nurse training, never worked at a hospital or trained or mentored a nurse and never wrote a book, article, pamphlet or sentence on nursing. The plaque in the Mary Seacole Building at Brunel University twice uses 'pioneer' in reference to her, without saying what she pioneered. Awards announced by the Department of Health and NHS Employers in 2013 named Seacole a 'pioneer' of health care.[96]

In calling for a Seacole monument, the then president of the Royal College of Nursing, Sylvia Denton, made the puzzling claim that Seacole 'against all odds...had an unshakable belief in the power of nursing to make a difference.' The article quoting her also errs in calling Seacole a 'pioneering nurse' awarded two medals and goes on to claim that she 'changed the face of modern nursing.'[97] How she changed it the author did not say. The deep belief that nursing can make a difference was Nightingale's and it was largely her work, and that of nurses she mentored, that changed the face of modern nursing.

The entry on Seacole in Rappaport's *Encyclopedia* asserts that Seacole's purpose in going to the Crimea was 'to pioneer the nursing of the sick and wounded' during the war and that she made a 'unique contribution to the development of nursing' (2:631), not specified. Seacole's memoir more modestly explained that she wanted to join the *second* contingent, having been too busy attending to her gold mining stocks to try for the first (*WA* 76). Robinson, in her biography, has Seacole 'managing a professional nursing

---

[96] Debbie Andalo, 'How to get ahead in...NHS leadership,' *Guardian* 8 May 2013.

[97] Carol Davis, 'Living Her Dream,' *Nursing Standard* 18,32 (21 April 2004):12.

service for the British Army' (72), although the British Army, pre-Nightingale, did not employ any professional nurses. The 'nurse practitioner' label appears in a public lecture at the Florence Nightingale Museum,'[98] while a history website makes her 'the first nurse practitioner.'[99] A doctoral thesis similarly uses 'first nurse practitioner,' crediting her with 'outstanding clinical skills' and 'positive patient outcomes.' Seacole may indeed have had the favourable patient outcomes and clinical skills claimed, but how would anyone know? There are no independent assessments of her diagnoses or remedies. That thesis also erroneously made her hut-store into 'a boarding house and clinic near the front lines.'[100]

Anionwu asserts that 'some nurses are angry that they were not taught about Mary Seacole alongside Florence Nightingale,'[101] as if they had made equal or even similar contributions. A *Nursing Standard* article holds that Seacole is a 'role model for every ethnic group' and should be 'routinely' taught in nursing education. But what would be taught? She herself admitted blunders and used toxic substances that she thought were effective at the time. The article further states that, in her day, Seacole was recognized 'in a similar way to Florence Nightingale.'[102] But this is not true either. Seacole was a celebrity, feted and cheered in public, which Nightingale was not. However, Nightingale was recognized for her work on nursing, hospital reform and health statistics. She was made a fellow of the Royal Statistical Society in 1858 (the first woman fellow) and named 'life governor' of

---

[98] Elizabeth Anionwu, 'The Nursing Practice of Mary Seacole: Influences, Case Studies and the Opinion of Others,' Public lecture, Florence Nightingale Museum 30 April 2012.

[99] Helen J. Seaton, 'Another Florence Nightingale: The Rediscovery of Mary Seacole,' English History from Victoria Web.

[100] Bonnie McKay Harmer, Silenced in History: A Historical Study of Mary Seacole abstract.

[101] Anionwu, *Short History* 35.

[102] Lynne Pearce, 'Tribute to a Visionary,' *Nursing Standard* 19,4 (6 October 2004):16–17.

several London teaching hospitals (beginning in 1856 with the London and St Mary's). She was celebrated, in her absence, at Crimean banquets, for example in Edinburgh, where more than 2,000 guests made toasts to 'the British Army, the Navy, our Allies, the Memory of those who fell, and Florence Nightingale.'[103] An electronic source calls Seacole's nursing skills 'undeniably...groundbreaking,' so that it would be insulting to call her the 'black Florence Nightingale.' But what were those skills and what ground did they break? This source also fictionalizes her travels, calling her a 'seeker of knowledge' who went 'to Cuba, Haiti, the Bahamas and Central America, learning all the while the best of conventional nursing skills that she would add to her own Creole.'[104] Yet Seacole herself gave entirely different purposes for those travels, for example, acquiring shells and shell work for sale from the Bahamas, not nursing knowledge or skills, and said nothing about seeking knowledge in any of these places (5).

Another web source holds that 'Mary Seacole changed the way that people thought about nursing forever,' linking her to (Nightingale's) 1860 establishment of 'Britain's first school for nursing' at St Thomas' Hospital. The website also mistakenly claims that Seacole ran a 'little hospital' over her store, where she 'cleaned wounds and applied bandages' and the usual battlefield exploits of treating soldiers 'while under gunfire.' According Seacole credit for the first nursing school also serves to justify the installation of her statue there.

Seacole's own statements about nursing are confined to a few occasions when she cared for someone at home. She called herself once 'doctress, nurse and "mother"' (124), once 'doctress and nurse' (125) and twice 'nurse and doctress' (7 and 127), in none of these cases a reference to hospital nursing. During the Crimean War, when she used the term 'nurse,' she was, without exception, referring to Nightingale or one of her nurses.

---

[103] 'The Edinburgh Crimean Banquet,' *The Times* 24 October 1856:7.

[104] Athena Krambides, 'Finding Mary Seacole in London,' *Culture* 24, 11 December 2006.

Yet a BBC video on Seacole in its Famous People series depicts her in a nurse's uniform at the bedside of a soldier, although she never wore a uniform at any time in her life and her Crimean 'patients' were relatively healthy walk-ins.

To boost Seacole's nursing credentials, some of her supporters effectively deny that Nightingale was a nurse at all. Ramdin, for example, confines her role at Scutari to being 'mainly administrative, although she did visit wards' (84). Hugh Small, in a BBC film, calls Nightingale a 'disembodied animal,' who lobbied rather than doing the real nursing.[105] A nurse commentator has Nightingale being 'more of a nurse administrator,' while Seacole 'was a true trauma nurse.'[106] Yet Nightingale did in fact do much hands-on nursing during the Crimean War. As to the 'true trauma nurse claim,' how can anyone know? Her 'patients' were all fit and some of the wounds she treated were from sports injuries when the war was effectively over. Anionwu claims Seacole was a 'hands-on' nurse, while Nightingale merely wrote letters.[107]

An article in a clinical nursing journal credits Seacole with an astonishing feat, that after making her own way to the Crimea to 'serve both the comfort and medical needs of the wounded soldiers,' she whipped back by night (300 miles by sea) to work 'side by side with Nightingale at Scutari as a volunteer nurse.' If this were true, she would well deserve being honoured, if not as 'one of the greatest women of all times,'[108] surely the speediest. Another source similarly has her both running her own hospital and, after 7 p.m., miraculously

---

[105] BBC Knowledge, 'Mary Seacole: A Hidden History,' 2000.

[106] Julie Santy and Chris Knight, 'Nurses in War,' *Journal of Orthopaedic Nursing* 12,1 (February 2008):51.

[107] Elizabeth Anionwu, 'What can Florence and Mary Teach us about Nursing Today?' *Nursing Standard* website.

[108] P.R. Messmer and Y. Parchment, 'Mary Grant Seacole: The First Nurse Practitioner,' *Clinical Excellence for Nurse Practitioners: The International Journal of NPACE* 2,1 (February 1998):47.

turning up as a volunteer at Nightingale's,[109] after which she would have to dash back the 300 miles in the morning to start cooking the day's meals for officers. An article in the *American Journal of Nursing*, which identified Seacole as a 'nursing leader,' has her nursing in the war 'with Florence Nightingale,' without citing amazing feats of self-propulsion.[110]

Some Seacole supporters go beyond mere mythologizing to attribute Nightingale's achievements to the new heroine. Rappaport's entry on Seacole is a good example, and makes one wonder why a staunch imperialist like Seacole who never proposed any social reform should be in an encyclopedia on social reformers in the first place. Yet the entry credits her, in the Crimea, with introducing 'methods of nursing that emphasized cleanliness, plenty of ventilation and an abundance of her own home-cooked food' (2:631), when it was Nightingale who worked assiduously to ensure cleanliness and improve food (in newly designed hospital kitchens, not home-cooked) and it took a whole sanitary commission to improve ventilation.

A *Nursing Standard* article which calls Seacole a 'military nurse' also, in effect, transfers Nightingale's work to her when it reports that Seacole (supposedly) confronted 'an ankle-deep "swamp of filth"' on the front line, with shallow graves and dying military animals.[111] But Seacole described nothing of the sort in her memoir and the scene rather evokes what Nightingale faced at the Barrack Hospital, related in Chapter 2 (p 60–61). 'Filth,' not so incidentally, was a code word for feces. The dying animals were in hospital sewers and drains, which Nightingale reported in her *Notes on the Health of the British Army*, using the official report of the Sanitary Commission (described in *CW*

---

[109] M. Elizabeth Carnegie, *The Path We Tread: Blacks in Nursing* 3.

[110] Fannie M. July, 'Can You Identify These Nursing Leaders?' *American Journal of Nursing* 19,2 (February 1990):66.

[111] Erin Dean, 'Campaign for Mary Seacole Memorial Is Stepped Up in the Face of Opposition,' *Nursing Standard* 24,34 (28 April 2010):12.

604 and 704–08). Those defects were not on the front line and not near Seacole at all.

The BBC Learning Zone item already cited in Myth 2 also promotes the pioneer myth, with the claim that Seacole devised 'new methods in nursing,' saving 'many lives' and setting up a 'rest home for soldiers.' Harriet Washington's foreword to *Wonderful Adventures* calls Seacole 'an uncommonly skilled nurse specializing in tropical diseases' and even 'much more than that' (xvii). Neither source gives concrete examples of the skills or the lives saved. An article in the oldest pan-African journal calls Seacole 'overqualified for the Crimea job.' Her testimonials came 'from notable doctors and British military officers' and her experience was 'light years' ahead of Nightingale's.[112]

When approving the use of its site for a Seacole statue, the Guy's and St Thomas' NHS Foundation Trust described her as 'Britain's black heroine who gave her life's work' in support of nursing's 'early development.'[113] But the person who gave her life's work to the early development of nursing was Nightingale.

The secretary of state for health in 1994, Brian Mawhinney, was so misinformed as to credit Seacole with having made a 'major contribution to nursing the wounded' in the Crimean War, then working 'as a nurse in and around London' as a contemporary of Nightingale's, altogether being 'an outstanding black British nurse.'[114] Yet, according to her own memoir, Seacole's first aid to the wounded in the Crimean War was confined to a number of hours and she is not known ever to have nursed anywhere in or around London.

The general secretary of the Royal College of Nursing, Peter Carter, thought that Seacole should be treated in 'equal measure' to Nightingale

---

[112] Ankomah Baffour, 'Mary Seacole — The Forgotten Nightingale: Part 2,' *New African* 389 (1 October 2000):34–38.

[113] Sorenson, 'Mary Seacole Memorial Statue Update.'

[114] Quoted in 'Mary Seacole Nursing Award Launched in the United Kingdom,' *Journal of Advanced Nursing* 20,2 (1994):207.

and Edith Cavell,[115] a nurse executed by the Germans for treason in World War I for helping British and French soldiers escape Belgium. Cavell certainly was a nurse — indeed she trained at a school where Nightingale mentored the matron and she served as night superintendent at a workhouse infirmary where Nightingale got professional nursing introduced. But Cavell is celebrated for her bravery and patriotism, not her nursing.

Two Bristol nurses are typical of many in arguing that International Nurses' Day, celebrated on Nightingale's birthday, should also 'acknowledge the contribution of other great nurses in history, such as Mary Seacole,' without saying what would constitute a great nurse or how Seacole qualified.[116] A *Nursing Times* article calls Seacole 'Nightingale's equal' and urges that she be recognized in schools of nursing and in histories of nursing in England, without saying what her equal contribution was.[117] Channel 4's 'Real Angel of the Crimea' calls Seacole 'a person of equal stature and significance' and her 'hotel' a hospital.

The National Portrait Gallery described Seacole's work as 'complementary' to that of Nightingale.[118] Nurses increasingly have taken up this theme of equal or equivalent contributions. Yet none of them has given any specifics as to what Seacole's contribution was, nor are any contributions evident (see the Timelime in Chapter 1).

War historian Clive Ponting insisted that Seacole 'achieved as much, if not more, for the British soldiers' as Nightingale,[119] although he did not say exactly what. A review of his book notes that he followed F.B.

---

[115] Petra Kendall-Rayner, 'Choice of Nightingale's "Shrine" for Seacole Memorial Contested,' *Nursing Standard* 21,34 (2 May 2007):8.

[116] Caroline Haines and Rebecca Hoskins, 'Celebrating Nursing,' *Paediatric Nursing* 20,6 (September 2008):36.

[117] Paul Crawford, 'The Other Lady with the Lamp,' *Nursing The Times* 88,11 (1992):58.

[118] National Portrait Gallery, 'Lost Portrait of Mary Seacole Discovered,' online 10 January 2005.

[119] Clive Ponting, *The Crimean War: The Truth behind the Myth* 202.

Smith's 'hostile biography' of Nightingale and failed to notice how she brought about 'systematic reform of the nursing profession.'[120]

A comparison of the two women on a webpage, while judging that Nightingale 'quite rightly earned immortality,' rates Seacole's worth more highly. She 'outshone' Nightingale, 'outmatched her in medical skills' and was 'more accomplished, more courageous' thanks to 'nursing skills' learned from her mother.[121] It gives no particulars on any of these claims.

Some commentators link Seacole with Nightingale, for example, Anionwu calls them two 'nursing luminaries.' She wonders how often they met and what they would have said to each other,[122] although the one recorded meeting between them (Seacole's) relates no discussion of nursing at all (*WA* 90–91). In another publication, the same author describes that meeting as the 'first' time they met, implying that there were others. She further calls them both 'good at networking,' both committed to holistic nursing practice, sanitation, nutrition and care during illness and death. Both women used 'their anger about poor nursing care to bring about change.'[123] Yet Anionwu provides no evidence of changes effected by Seacole to nursing care. In another article, Anionwu calls Seacole 'a pioneer, as Florence Nightingale was,'[124] without stating what Seacole pioneered. Her use of mercury chloride and lead acetate in remedies (*WA* 31) might have been pioneering for nurses, but both poisonous substances were commonly used by doctors at the time.

---

[120] Ferdinand Mount, 'Lord Cardigan's Cherry Pants,' *London Review of Books* (20 May 2004):10.

[121] Baker, 'Forgotten War Nurse.'

[122] Anionwu, *Short History* 29.

[123] Elizabeth Anionwu, 'A History that Lives on,' *Nursing Standard* 26,5 (5 October 2011):18.

[124] Elizabeth Anionwu, 'Mary Seacole: Nursing Care in Many Lands,' *British Journal of Healthcare Assistants* 6,5 (May 2012):244.

Myth 8: Seacole more than a nurse — a doctor and pharmacist

For some commentators, being a pioneer or celebrated nurse is not enough. According to Dr Richard Grant, senior lecturer at the University of Luton, Seacole was not only a 'brilliant nurse,' but a 'very good doctor' and 'very intelligent pharmacist.' He calls her remedies 'far in advance' of British medicine at the time, although he mentions not a one in the interview he gave for the BBC film. Unhappily, Seacole followed the worst practices of medicine of the time, adding toxic substances such as mercury chloride and acetate of lead to her remedies. Grant fails to specify anything more about the 'powerful Caribbean and African remedies' which, he says, she employed,[125] nor did Seacole give the names of any in her memoir. Management consultant Hugh Small, interviewed in the same film, holds that 'she was in fact what we would call now a general practitioner.' A broadcast on BBC Woman's Hour called her 'Medical Pioneer.'[126]

An open letter to the secretary of state for education credited Seacole with delivering 'holistic care to the wounded of all nations' during the war, making her 'a sort of one-person Red Cross,' and even 'developing new approaches to health care.'[127]

A foundation school history website adds qualifications in midwifery to those of being 'an influential nurse' and, like Nightingale, an improver of public health.[128] The Royal College of Nursing website credits Seacole with learning midwifery, along with herbal medicines, from her

---

[125] BBC Knowledge, 'Mary Seacole: A Hidden History,' first broadcast in September 2000. An email to Dr Grant requesting specifics went unanswered.

[126] Radio 4, 10 February 2004.

[127] Jeanette Arnold, OBE, open letter to Michael Gove 31 January 2013, Labour List.

[128] History Dept., Folkestone School for Girls, Revision Guide: Medicine Through Time. Accessed 24 April 2013.

mother,[129] although she never mentioned herself or her mother learning or practising midwifery in her memoir. A *Nursing Times* article also erroneously adds midwifery to her skills.[130] Another source calls her a 'born healer,'[131] with an exaggerated working schedule, 'serving breakfast to off-duty troops, caring for the sick and wounded able to make their own way to her hut, visiting the military hospital with books and papers, mending torn uniforms' (249–50).

The *Nursing Standard* article which credits Seacole with changing the face of modern nursing also has her travelling the world to add European medical knowledge to her 'traditional skills.'[132] Certainly her memoir made no such claim, nor gave any specifics of what her herbal remedies were, nor where she might have acquired European medical knowledge.

An editorial defines 'doctress' as 'a woman doctor who, though not formally trained, was "well versed with the prognosis and treatment of tropical diseases, general ailments and wounds," often administering her own remedies of herbs and local plants.'[133] That Seacole added harmful substances to her remedies was not mentioned. A children's book has Seacole as a 'nurse practitioner' carrying out treatments usually done only by doctors.[134]

Washington's error-prone foreword calls Seacole 'the only trained medical professional' at Cruces, Panama (xiii), adding that she 'sought out perilous situations and...cut the Gordian knot by boldly undertaking private practice without waiting for license' (xvii). She:

---

[129] Royal College of Nursing. Website. Mary Seacole (1805–1881) accessed October 2013.

[130] Catharine Watson, 'Hidden From History,' *Nursing The Times* 80,41 (1984):16.

[131] Peter Fryer, 'Mary Seacole' 246.

[132] Carol Davis, 'Living Her Dream,' *Nursing Standard* 18,32 (21 April 2004):12.

[133] James P. Smith, 'Mary Jane Seacole 1805–1881: A Black British Nurse,' *Journal of Advanced Nursing* 9,5 (1984):427.

[134] Brian Williams, *The Life and World of Mary Seacole* 29.

did more to expand the horizons of women in medicine than some of her contemporaries who remain household names. Every midwife, nurse practitioner and woman doctor practising today owes Seacole's pioneering soul a great debt (xii).

Author Eric Huntley stated that Seacole worked 'along with European doctors' when she developed a medicine which cured yellow fever and cholera (43), a point already disputed during the discussion of successful cures. She did not mention working along with any doctor, any more than she claimed those cures.

One website has Seacole spending her married life travelling, with her husband, in 'the other islands of the Caribbean,' where she 'continued to develop her healing skills, learning the practices and cures native to the islands she visited.'[135] In fact the couple ran a store in Black River, Jamaica (5) and her memoir mentions no travels with him, nor developing healing skills in her own Caribbean travels.

A children's book with Seacole wearing a nurse's uniform on the cover is also wrong on nearly everything in the text. Her mother, it says, was a 'doctor' and she wanted to be one too when she grew up.[136] A foundation geared at social innovation has both Nightingale and Seacole setting up medical facilities in the war (Seacole's are identified as 'new medical facilities'); it describes Seacole as a 'faith-inspired pioneer.'[137] But it was Nightingale who was inspired by faith and, while she hardly set up any medical facilities, she did a great deal to improve care, while Seacole was running her business.

The purportedly factual introduction to a novel on Seacole gives, as the intention for the projected Seacole statue, 'to preserve in history the many contributions she made to health care and to the military field

---

[135] Lynda Osborne, 'The Life of Mary Seacole: Unknown Angel of the Crimean War,' *Historical Biographies* suite 101, 28 July 2009.

[136] Castor, *Mary Seacole* 6.

[137] Young Foundation, *Social Silicon Valleys: A Manifesto for Social Innovation* 12.

services,'[138] not one of which it specified, nor do any appear in her memoir. What military field services?

Anionwu contrasts the two women on their relations with doctors: Nightingale was 'controlling' and 'clashed with many doctors,' while Seacole 'generally got on well with her medical colleagues,'[139] yet Seacole is not known to have had any contact with army doctors post-Crimea and only one doctor (in the navy) is on the list of contributors to the funds raised for her. There is no evidence that any doctor treated her as a medical colleague at any time. A doctor who served with the Turkish forces in the Crimea called her 'a sutler who kept a store at Kadikoi, two or three miles from British headquarters.'[140] A surgeon in the Crimea described her as 'one of the many sutlers or camp followers who sold goods (mostly food and drink) to the troops, and who followed the army on every campaign, appearing in the most unlikely places.'[141] Seacole herself acknowledged that the tea and lemonade she served soldiers on the wharf waiting transport to Scutari was 'all the doctors would allow me to give' (101), which hardly suggests 'collegial' relations.

There is no doubt that some doctors did not like Nightingale or her women nurses, but overall their fears were allayed and they came to accept the nurses' presence. A number of later Crimean War doctors became Nightingale's colleagues for years later working on nursing, hospital and health care reform: Dr John Sutherland, head of the Sanitary Commission; Sir John McNeill, a doctor and head of the Supply Commission; and Dr E.A. Parkes, head of the civil hospital at Renkioi, later professor of military hygiene at Netley Hospital.

---

[138] S. Marie Vernon, Review, in Julia Buss, *Black Nightingale: Mary Seacole, Hero of the Crimean War*.

[139] Elizabeth Anionwu, 'A History that Lives on,' *Nursing Standard* 26,5 (5 October 2011):18.

[140] Buzzard, *With the Turkish Army in the Crimea* 179.

[141] Victor Bonham Carter, ed., *Surgeon in the Crimea* 192.

To buttress the claim of being 'more than a nurse,' some cite Seacole's supposed special relationship with Dr (later Sir) John Hall, inspector general of hospitals and principal medical officer in the Crimea. Seacole included in her memoir the following letter, dated 30 June 1856, which she represented as being from him and which most commentators take as authentic:

> She [Mary Seacole], not only from the knowledge she had acquired in the West Indies, was enabled to administer appropriate remedies for their ailments, but what was of as much importance, she charitably furnished them with proper nourishment, which they had no means of obtaining except in the hospital, and most of that class had an objection to go into hospital (129–30).

No such letter, however, can be found in Hall's papers[142] or at the War Office, where official letters were copied and docketed, or in S.M. Mitra's *The Life and Letters of Sir John Hall.* No one seems to have considered how unlikely it would have been for Hall to acknowledge publicly the lack of 'proper nourishment' available to soldiers or the need for charity to supply it. Officers of the Army Medical Department consistently held that ample provision had been made, so that charity was not needed. Yet this purported letter is used in fundraising for the Seacole Appeal.[143]

This dubious letter is cited as if it were genuine also by Alexander and Dewjee in the Introduction to their edition of *Wonderful Adventures* (10). Robinson also fell for it in her biography (142), although she was sceptical about Seacole winning medals. The letter serves nicely to score points against Nightingale.

Some Seacole supporters have gone even further by claiming that Hall inspected Seacole's bag of medicines and gave his sanction to her prescribing them. Seacole herself never said as much — and surely she

---

[142] His journal with copied letters is at the Wellcome Trust, Ms 8520.

[143] Anionwu, 'Mary Seacole: Nursing Care in Many Lands,' *British Journal of Healthcare Assistants* 6,5 (May 2012):248; Unison also quotes the letter: 'The Mary Seacole (1805–1880) Campaign "Turn her into Stone,"' 16//1/10.

would have had bragging rights if he had. The source for this claim is a supposed note of a conversation that Nightingale had with her sister, uncovered by Bostridge in papers at Claydon House. But the comment is merely a jotting in a lined book, with numerous others, all undated, on many subjects. In this one, Nightingale is referred to in the third person, which suggests that someone else said it:

> Dr Hall looked over her [Seacole's] medicine chest and gave her his sanction to prescribe — to mark the difference with F., in that he extended his protection to Seacole and opposed F. to his utmost.[144]

It is difficult to imagine the principal medical officer giving a person with no formal medical qualifications the same right to prescribe as his own officers, all of whom were qualified in medicine or surgery. Certainly Hall opposed Nightingale and her nurses, but that is not necessarily to his credit: he and Nightingale differed on the use of chloroform — she for it, he against — and most significantly on the adequacy of the hospitals — he inspected and approved the Turkish barrack, while she spoke out on how bad it was. Nightingale was hardly the only person to be critical of Hall: Lord Raglan, notably, censured him for the poor treatment of the men in transit to Scutari.[145] Dr Reid in his war letters called Hall a 'benevolent despot,' siding with Nightingale, not Hall, on the need for cleaning up the hospitals.[146]

Hall's dislike of Nightingale is set out frequently in his journal, along with his fondness for her adversary, the mother superior of the Irish Sisters of Mercy, Mary Francis Bridgeman. Bridgeman was agreeably uncomplaining, although her hospital at Koulali had the worst sanitary conditions and the highest death rate of all the war hospitals. Yet her

---

[144] Claydon House bundle 110; comment in Bostridge, *Florence Nightingale: The Woman and her Legend* 274.

[145] General order 13 December 1854, in *General Orders Issued to the Army of the East* 78; and on Raglan's general disapproval see Hibbert, *The Destruction of Lord Raglan* 210–14.

[146] Reid, *Soldier-Surgeon* 19.

writing shows no awareness of any problems — no wonder Hall liked her![147] His private journal, the *Life and Letters*, includes correspondence with a number of other nurses, but no mention of Seacole.

Myth 9: 'Black nurse,' 'black heroine'

There is a demand for more black heroes and heroines to be role models for the sizable black population in Britain. Since many blacks, especially Jamaicans, work in hospitals, the idea of a black nurse who was also a war heroine is appealing. The National Health Service is the largest employer of blacks in Britain.

A major difficulty, however, is the fact that Seacole herself was only one quarter black, a quadroon in the language of the time, and did not at all identify with her African roots — the words 'Africa' and 'African' do not appear in her memoir. There are good historical reasons for this distancing, which have been amply discussed elsewhere.[148] Biographer Robinson said that Seacole chose to 'ignore' her black ancestry, even using the prejudicial term 'nigger,' then pervasive. Seacole 'used prejudice as a weapon of self-defence' (173).

To counter the fiction that Seacole was black, essential for her being a black heroine or a black nurse, we have only to look at her own published

---

[147] For a particularly obsequious letter see Bridgeman's to Hall 10 April [1855], Add Mss 39867 f109. For more of Bridgeman's correspondence see Luddy, *Crimean Journals* 165–67, 180–81, 185–86, 188–90, 227–28, 229, 241–42

[148] See especially William L. Andrews, Introduction, *Wonderful Adventures* xxvii-xxxiv; Ziggi Alexander and Audrey Dewjee, Introduction, *Wonderful Adventures* 9–45; Jessica Howell, 'Mrs Seacole Prescribes Hybridity: Constitutional and Maternal Rhetoric in *Wonderful Adventures of Mrs Seacole in Many Lands*,' *Victorian Literature and Culture* 38,1 (2010):107–25; Sandra Pouchet Paquet, 'West Indian Autobiographical Consciousness in "The Wonderful Adventures of Mrs Seacole in Many Lands,"' *African American Review* 26 (1992):651–63; Rupprecht, 'Wonderful Adventures', in Lambert and Lester, eds, *Colonial Lives Across the British Empire* 176–201.

views. She was light-skinned, married to a white man, had a white business partner and served a white clientele. She described herself as being 'yellow,' the term then used for a fair complexion. Her references to her Creole roots were brief and negative (1–2).

As noted in Chapter 3, 'blacks' appear frequently as Seacole's employees, both in Panama and Crimea. 'Negroes' and 'niggers' also appear, again always in reference to other people. In Panama, Seacole had a black maid (39) and another black servant (12 and 36), both of whom were with her also in the Crimea. At her business in Panama, she employed a black barber (37), whom she called a 'grinning black' (38). Her brother at his hotel employed a black doorman (19) and black cooks (21), whom she called the 'excited nigger cooks' (20). Numerous other blacks, including some exemplary former slaves, appear in the Panama material.

At her hut in the Crimea, Seacole employed two black cooks, whom she also called her 'good-for-nothing black cooks' (141). Another servant was 'Jew Johnny' (92, 104, 109 and 113). Greeks in *Wonderful Adventures* were 'craven,' 'villainous-looking' (106) and 'cunning-eyed' (86), while Turks were 'the degenerate descendants of the fierce Arabs' (106), who were 'deliberate, slow and indolent' (109). Some of her racial references were gruesome, notably her description of roasted monkey 'whose grilled head bore a strong resemblance to a negro baby's,' while a piece in a monkey stew 'closely resembled a brown baby's limb' (69).

Few people who knew Seacole called her 'black.' Evelyn Wood is an exception, referring to her as 'an old black woman.'[149] Artist William Simpson calls her an 'elderly mulatto' (57), while Dr Reid uses 'mulatto' (44) or 'coloured woman' (13) in his *Soldier-Surgeon*. A story on the bankruptcy court refers to her as 'a lady of colour,' a flattering story awarding her four medals.[150] Another *Times* story notes the 'fine mahogany hue of the warm-hearted West Indian.'[151]

---

[149] Wood, *The Crimea in 1854 and 1894* 294.

[150] 'Bankruptcy Court: In re Seacole and Day,' *The Times* 7 November 1856 9A.

[151] From our special correspondent, 'The British Army,' *The Times* 16 May 1856 10D.

Yet the 'black' descriptor appears frequently in titles and subtitles. Robinson's biography was originally subtitled *The Black Woman Who Invented Modern Nursing* when announced by Carroll & Graf in 2004, but when it was came out it was *The Most Famous Black Woman of the Victorian Age* (Basic Books, 2004). The English edition's subtitle is *The Charismatic Black Nurse Who Became a Heroine of the Crimea* (Constable, 2005). A review of the biography necessarily uses the 'charismatic black nurse' wording.[152]

The BBC's 'Famous People' video calls Seacole a proper 'black nurse' who saved lives, while demonizing Nightingale as a white racist. A song in its Horrible Histories says it in dialect:

Me apply for Florence's crew.

She turn me down because me black....

Me nursed right upon de battlefield.

While Florence worked far from de war.

The original print version of Horrible Histories, however, did not make these errors.

Salih, in her Introduction to *Wonderful Adventures*, concedes that Seacole never said anything about slave revolts or the abolition of slavery in Jamaica and concludes that she displayed 'troublingly superior attitudes towards black people' (xxiii), although she did admire slaves who got away and made successful lives for themselves in Panama (xxvii). Racial prejudice was more openly expressed at the time, but Nightingale did not use racial slurs.

One tribute, which repeats many of the myths, acknowledges that Seacole was 'ultra-patriotic, imperialist and ambivalent about her own colour,' crediting her 'good Scotch blood' for her notable deeds and calling herself 'yellow' or 'brown,' although 'she called black people "niggers."' Overall, 'she endorsed Victorian British stereotypes.'[153]

---

[152] 'A Warm Portrait of Mary Seacole,' *Nursing Standard* 19,25 (2 March 2005):28.

[153] Angus Calder, *Gods, Mongrels and Demons* 330.

Several authors think that Seacole's contributions were devalued on account of her race. Novelist Salman Rushdie said as much in *The Satanic Verses*, quoted in Chapter 1. In her Introduction to *Wonderful Adventures*, Salih similarly complains that, while Seacole was a 'cause celebre' in Britain in the 1850s, she was 'rapidly obscured from view by the metaphorical glare of Florence Nightingale's candle' (xv). Jamaican-born nurse, the late Connie Mark, echoed the sentiment, if not the fiery metaphor, in explaining why Seacole, but not Nightingale, was forgotten after the Crimean War: why would you praise a black when you can praise a white woman?[154] She acknowledged no differences in the contributions of Seacole and Nightingale.

Washington's foreword to *Wonderful Adventures* holds that Seacole's contribution was obscured by 'racial' misunderstandings and that the black Nightingale comparison did Seacole an 'injustice' (xvii). It, however, gives not one instance of Seacole making a contribution to medicine or nursing, nor acknowledges her use of racist language.

Lord Soley, chair of the Seacole Statue Appeal Campaign, said that Seacole 'deserved to be remembered in the same way as Florence Nightingale,' without documenting any comparable contribution. This had not happened, he said, because Seacole was black.[155] Public health minister Anne Milton told the audience of a Seacole awards event that Seacole had been turned away from volunteering at 'one of history's bloodiest wars...because of her colour.' She knew of no story 'of more courage, dedication and passion' than Seacole's.[156]

---

[154] BBC Knowledge, 'Mary Seacole: A Hidden History.'

[155] 'Star Backs Seacole Statue Push,' *Nursing Standard* 8,43 (7 July 2004):9.

[156] 'An Inspiration: The Mary Seacole Awards,' *Community Practitioner* 84,12 (December 2011):4.

Myth 10: Rejection of Seacole as a nurse for the Crimea and later

One of the many faults Seacole supporters attribute to Nightingale is her supposed opposition to their heroine. As Chapter 3 has shown in detail, Nightingale did not refuse to employ Seacole in London, but indeed had already left for the war when Seacole made up her mind to go. Nor did she refuse to employ her when they met briefly at the Barrack Hospital in Scutari, the only account of which is Seacole's (78, 85, 89–91). Yet writer A.N. Wilson contends Nightingale rejected Seacole's service 'on racialist grounds.'[157] A book on the 'literary representation of war' similarly blames Nightingale for not recruiting Seacole to her nursing service due to 'racial prejudice.'[158] The Facebook site for the Mary Seacole Memorial Statue Appeal states: 'She faced racism from Florence Nightingale and the nursing elite.'

A New Zealand publication claims Seacole twice applied to go to the war, but was declined because of 'racism,' at which point readers are invited to reflect 'on the part Florence Nightingale played in this refusal.' But why should anyone 'reflect' when there is clear evidence that Nightingale played no such part? The article further minimizes the dangers Nightingale faced, while inventing dangers for Seacole, bullets 'whizzing' around her head 'while she did her job.'[159]

Rappaport's entry on Seacole in her *Encyclopedia* accuses Nightingale and the War Office of rejecting her for reasons of race (2:631). But Seacole's own memoir is clear that Nightingale had

---

[157] A.N. Wilson, *The Victorians* 178.

[158] Kate McLoughlin, *Authoring War: The Literary Representation of War from the Iliad* 32.

[159] Chris Cottingham, 'Signifying Mary: Move Over Florence — Nursing Has a New Mother. Well Guerilla Nursing That Is and It's Mrs Mary Seacole,' *Kai Tiaki: Nursing New Zealand* 17,5 (June 2011):5.

already left when she decided she wanted to go also (74). Months later, when Seacole saw her at Scutari, she sought a bed for the night and was given one. By then she was no longer looking for a job as she had a business partner waiting for her at Balaclava and supplies en route (Rappaport never mentions the business partner or the business plan and purchases).

A book on the 'misadventures of military history' makes the usual errors of claiming that Nightingale refused to receive Seacole in London, 'for reasons that can only be conjectured,' and then turned her away 'once again' in Turkey.[160] An article based on a doctoral dissertation has her refused four times (although without mention of race) by British officials and by Nightingale, who is described as 'the young novice nurse' appointed to head the nursing services. Along with many of the usual errors about Seacole's experience and competence, the article also has her becoming 'an advocate for the needs of war widows and orphans,' activities she never mentioned[161] but which were concerns of Nightingale's for decades after the war.

The website Science Museum: Exploring the History of Medicine, after incorrectly stating that Nightingale never met Seacole (they probably met for five minutes), says that she was 'hostile' to Seacole both throughout the war and after, for being a 'single woman' who sold alcohol (Seacole was a widow). Nightingale was not pleased with men or women, of any marital status, selling alcohol to soldiers, who were given 5 oz of rum a day as part of their rations.

A discussion of Seacole as a travel writer recounts the usual errors of her being refused as a nurse by Nightingale,[162] expressing much resentment that Seacole did not acquire the same reputation. Further,

---

[160] Donald, *Loose Cannons: 101 Myths* 66.

[161] Bonnie Harmer, 'Women in History — Mary Seacole,' *Journal of Women in Educational Leadership* 3,2 (4 January 2005):83–84.

[162] Cheryl J. Fish, 'Travelling Medicine Chest: Mary Seacole "Plays Doctor" at Colonial Crossroads in Panama and in the Crimea,' 65.

her memoir is described as a 'counternarrative to the white, Western myth of Florence Nightingale' (2). Nightingale, 'that Victorian "ministering angel"' is then faulted for having made only 'slight mention of Seacole in her Crimean letters, expressing disapproval' (66), when in fact she made no mention of Seacole in those letters at all — the author provides no examples.

In the Channel 4 film, 'Mary Seacole: The Real Angel of the Crimea,' the putdown of Nightingale is obvious in the title. Nightingale and Seacole are contrasted in the film, always to the advantage of the latter: Nightingale 'ruled with an iron hand,' while Seacole did 'hands-on work.' Nightingale 'did not touch' soldiers, it imaginatively asserts — how did they know? Surveillance cameras in the Barrack Hospital? One soldier (as portrayed by an actor) uttered resentfully that they 'could only kiss her shadow.' Really? Soldiers with contagious diseases should have kissed her?

In Horrible Histories, a white Florence Nightingale, dressed in a nurse's uniform — this is quite realistic, although not the exact uniform she wore — elbows aside a black Seacole, also dressed in a nurse's uniform, although she never wore one. Nightingale could not have elbowed her out of the way, even if she had wanted to.

Soyer's reports of the relationship between the two women in his *Culinary Campaign* belie the rejection myth. He and Seacole discussed Nightingale together on several occasions, each time positively (233 and 434). He also reports Seacole telling him that 'she had spent a few days with Miss Nightingale' (300), which must be wrong, for the only meeting in her memoir was the brief one at Scutari. He reports Nightingale's commendation of Seacole for doing good for 'the poor soldiers' (436).

Some commentators claim Nightingale not only rejected Seacole at the start of the Crimean War, but carried on her hostility as late as the Franco-Prussian War in 1870. The contention is that Seacole offered to go to that war — for what purpose is not mentioned. She conveyed this to Sir Harry Verney, a vice-president of the National Aid Society and Nightingale's brother-in-law. Nightingale is then said to have seen to it that Seacole's offer was spurned. The *Oxford Companion to Black*

British History similarly makes the point of a rejected offer, also claiming that Seacole was turned down for the Indian Mutiny.[163] But what was the offer — catering or nursing? The British were not belligerents in that war, which took place when Seacole was sixty-five and had been retired for years.

A catering operation for French or German officers could not have worked anyway, for the British Army in the Crimea was stationary for a year and a half before Sebastopol, while armies in the Franco-Prussian War moved. Seacole could hardly have offered any food service to officers akin to that she provided the British in the Crimea. She also spoke neither French nor German.

The possibility of sending British nurses to the Franco-Prussian War was considered early on and Nightingale herself answered applicants' letters and forwarded them, with comments, to the National Aid Society.[164] It soon became clear, however, that neither of the belligerents wanted British nurses (they had enough of their own). Nightingale recommended only one: Florence Lees, who went, at the request of the crown princess, to her hospital in Prussia. Lees was already nursing in France when the war broke out and spoke both French and German.[165]

The letter Nightingale wrote Sir Harry about Seacole is reproduced here (his to her, if there was one, is not extant). Seacole campaigners describe it as an attack on her reputation, although the letter was private and remained so for at least a century after Seacole's death. Obviously it was not burned, as Nightingale intended.

---

[163] Jane Robinson, 'Seacole, Mary Jane (c1805–1881),' in David Dabydeen, et al., eds, *Oxford Companion to Black British History* online source.

[164] McDonald, ed., *Florence Nightingale on Wars and the War Office* 632–35 and 640–81.

[165] Florence Lees, 'In a Fever Hospital Before Metz' and 'The Crown Princess's Lazareth for the Wounded,' *Good Words* (1873):322–28 and 500–05.

From: Nightingale letter to Sir Harry Verney, Wellcome Trust Ms 9004/60

5 August 1870

Burn. Mrs Seacole. I dare say you know more about her.... She kept
— I will not call it a 'bad house,'[166] but something not very unlike it
— in the Crimean War. She was very kind to the men and, what is
more, to the officers — and did some good — and made many drunk.
(A shameful or ignorant imposture was practised on the queen, who
subscribed to the 'Seacole Testimonial.')

I had the greatest difficulty in repelling Mrs Seacole's advances
and in preventing association between her and my nurses (absolutely
out of the question) when we established two hospitals nursed by us
between Kadikoi and the 'Seacole establishment' (in the Crimea). But
I was successful — without any open collision with Mrs Seacole,
which I was anxious to avoid. (You will understand that any 'rivalry'
between the 'Seacole' and the 'Nightingale' 'establishment' was very
much to be averted.)

Anyone who employs Mrs Seacole will introduce much kindness
— also much drunkenness and improper conduct, wherever she is.
She had then, however, one or more 'persons' with her, whom (I
conclude) she has not now. I conclude (and believe) that respectable
officers were entirely ignorant of what I could not help knowing, as a
matron and chaperone and mother of the army.//

The publisher's description of Robinson's biography turned Nightingale's
measured statement above into condemnation of Seacole as 'a brothel-
keeping quack,' words she nowhere used.

An article including analysis of Seacole's 'hybridity,' or mixed-
race background, repeats the accusation that Nightingale treated
Seacole badly and was 'unequivocally negative' to Seacole's 'petition'

---

[166] A reference the availability of prostitutes, commonly part of the business of
public houses or taverns.

to nurse the wounded in the Franco-Prussian war.[167] But where and what was this petition? Sir Harry Verney evidently asked Nightingale something about Seacole, but there is nothing to suggest that she ever applied to become a nurse.

Seacole supporters make much of a statement supposed to have been made by Nightingale to her sister, but for which the source is but another undated pencil jotting — seventeen words — in the lined book already cited: 'Mrs Seacole, woman of bad character, kept a bad house. Daughter about fourteen her child of Colonel Bunbury.'[168] There is nothing in Nightingale's own hand to suggest that she ever said this, and the information, or gossip, could have come from any number of people who had visited the Crimea.

Growth of the myths

The medals myth alone goes back to Seacole herself. She began wearing medals in London in November 1856, at her first bankruptcy hearing. Dr Reid later saw her wearing them while walking in Charing Cross (recounted in Chapter 3). She had her portrait painted by Challen in 1869 wearing three medals, her bust sculpted by Gleichen in 1871 with four medals and a photograph taken for a carte de visite in 1873, when she went back to three medals.

Contemporary accounts of Seacole were routinely positive, but fall far short of heroism. War correspondent Russell, the most generous in his tribute, called her 'the good old woman' who brought plum pudding on the day of the last assault at the Redan.[169] She gave the 'last offices,'

---

[167] Jessica Howell, 'Mrs Seacole Prescribes Hybridity: Constitutional and Maternal Rhetoric in *Wonderful Adventures of Mrs Seacole in Many Lands*,' *Victorian Literature and Culture* 38,1 (2010):107–25.

[168] Jottings in Parthenope Nightingale's hand, Claydon House bundle 110.

[169] From our own correspondent, 'The British Army,' *The Times* 16 May 1856 10C.

closing the eyes of dying or dead soldiers, but never said that she saved thousands, or any. She was a 'sutler' who 'redeemed' the profession from its reputation of 'plunder' and gave 'aid and succour.'[170] In his letter to the editor on fundraising soon after, Russell hoped that people would be 'liberal and kind' in their response,[171] again stressing her kindness, not heroics.

Even the incorrect *The Times* report that claimed Seacole had been awarded medals attributed them to her kindness to the soldiers, not bravery.[172] A letter to the newspaper just after that boosted the sentiment to 'bountiful kindness.'[173] Seacole's friend Alexis Soyer, in his 1857 memoir, refers to her 'benevolent exertions.' He also calls her 'celebrated' and 'illustrious' (232 and 482), but not heroic. Dr Reid, in his memoir, refers to her 'kindness to the wounded and sick awaiting evacuation at Balaclava' (44), when she gave out tea, cake and lemonade. By contrast, he accords a whole chapter to Nightingale's work, which he judged to have resulted in great improvements. Dr Lawson refers to Seacole acting 'out of the goodness of her heart.'[174] A *Lancet* story supporting fundraising for her in 1867 calls her a 'kind-hearted, good creature,' who gave 'generous service' on horseback with her preservatives.[175] A chaplain to the Naval Brigade in the Crimea praised her for her 'deeds of mercy,' again without mentioning heroism or medals, but paid more attention to the improvements Nightingale and the Sanitary Commission brought about.[176]

---

[170] Russell, 'To the Reader,' Seacole, *Wonderful Adventures* viii.

[171] W.H.R., letter to the editor, 'The Seacole Fund,' *The Times* 11 April 1857 8D.

[172] 'Bankruptcy Court: In re Seacole and Day,' *The Times* 7 November 1856 9A.

[173] 'Mrs Seacole,' *The Times* 28 November 1856 8A.

[174] Bonham Carter, ed., *Surgeon in the Crimea* 157.

[175] 'Mrs Seacole,' *The Lancet* (9 February 1867):182.

[176] Mrs Tom Kelly and Samuel Kelson Stothert, *From the Fleet in the Fifties* 161–62 on Seacole, Chapter 21 on Nightingale.

Obituaries on Seacole's death in 1881 circulated statements verging on heroism. The one in *The Times*, quoted in Chapter 3 (p 108), was wildly inaccurate. It had Seacole risking her life at 'many' battles, but still it did not mention her being awarded any medals.

The term 'bravery' seems to have been first applied to Seacole in a 1903 book on heroic women, which gave generous praise both to Nightingale and Seacole. The latter was described as 'another woman, working apart from Miss Nightingale,' who 'performed deeds of bravery and humanity.' There are a number of exaggerations and several of the usual errors, but, even with the praise, there was nothing about medals.[177]

A *Times* story in 1954, on the centenary of the start of the Crimean War, added fresh inaccuracies and exaggerations. Still, it mentioned no medals and its final words celebrated Seacole's 'determination and humanity,'[178] which are undeniable, not heroics.

A 1970 book asserted most of the myths (successful cures, rejection by Nightingale, hotel with a top storey for hospital stays, services to wounded soldiers, time on the battlefield), but still without claims of vast numbers saved, and only one medal.[179]

A major change came in 1984 on the first reissue of *Wonderful Adventures*, with an Introduction that set out core misinformation: Seacole's supposed management of British Army nursing in Kingston, providing 'excellent medical supervision,' being a 'skilful surgeon' herself (17), routinely riding out to the battlefield (25), gaining the approbation of Sir John Hall (26) and then being given medals (35). Only two years later this reissue was praised in a nursing history journal for its 'carefully researched introduction.'[180] The campaign to replace

---

[177] Henry Charles Moore, *Noble Deeds of the World's Heroines*.

[178] 'Mrs Seacole: A West Indian Nurse in the Crimea,' *The Times* 24 December 1954 8E.

[179] Piers Compton, *Colonel's Lady and Camp Follower: The Story of Women in the Crimean War*.

[180] James P. Smith, 'Mary Jane Seacole 1805–1881: A Black British Nurse,' *Journal of Advanced Nursing* 9,5 (September 1984):428.

Nightingale with Seacole is much more recent, beginning in the early twenty-first century with the launch of the Seacole statue campaign.

Falsifying history and creating myths requires, along with the embellishment and invention of exploits for the hero or heroine, a studied silence about facts that contradict the narrative. Seacole campaigners simply do not quote her acknowledgment of 'lamentable blunders' in remedies or mention her taking loot from the bodies of Russians and Russian churches. Her frequent racial slurs are ignored by most commentators. The longer extracts provided in Chapter 6 reintroduce these omitted passages, in her own words, in context. They also permit a better look at *Wonderful Adventures* itself, which remains a real achievement whether fully written by Seacole or 'as told to' the editor.

Chapter 6

Mary Seacole in her own words

Seacole's purpose in publishing *Wonderful Adventures of Mrs Seacole in Many Lands* was undoubtedly practical: to raise cash. She had been declared bankrupt in April 1857 and her brief attempt at running a store at Aldershot had promptly failed. How much, if any, of the book she actually wrote is not known. There is no surviving manuscript or any correspondence with the publisher or the editor, W.J.S., listed on the title page. Biographer Robinson, who identified the editor as W.J. Stewart, thought that Seacole might have dictated it to him (168). Certainly the book reads with the directness of the spoken voice. War correspondent W.H. Russell wrote a highly complimentary two-page 'Introductory Preface,' making points that would be used to fundraise for Seacole and which continue to be cited by Seacole supporters today. Details of translations and later major editions are given in the References.

Wonderful Adventures is frequently called an 'autobiography' but 'travel memoir' would be more accurate, whether it is a regularly authored book or 'as told to.' Normal biographical material is simply missing, such as the subject's date of birth and schooling, her father's name and occupation (other than soldier) and his role in the family or date of death. Seacole's married life is recounted in ten lines, the first twenty-five years of her life takes up a mere twenty-five of a total 200 pages. There is no mention of the daughter who, according to Alexis Soyer, lived with her in the Crimea. The book ends when Seacole is only fifty-one years old. Most of it (twelve chapters) is about the Crimean period.

If *Wonderful Adventures* is no autobiography, it is successful as a travel memoir. The writing is lively, the characters and stories compelling, especially the accounts of the Panamanian route to the California Gold Rush and then the Crimea. Memoirs, journals and letters from the Crimean War exist in vast quantities, but Seacole's perspective was distinctive and she told her story well. Her *Wonderful Adventures* not only entertains and amuses, but describes and interprets other societies as the best travel literature does. It established Seacole's reputation as a traveller and put her into a distinguished group of women travel writers: Lady Mary Wortley Montagu, for her *Turkish Letters*, published posthumously in 1764; Harriet Martineau for her *Society in America*, 1837; and Flora Tristan for *Perigrinations of a Pariah* (on Peru), 1837 and *Promenades in London*, 1840, to give a few examples. Nightingale's *Letters from Egypt*, relating her trip up and down the Nile, were printed (for private circulation) in 1854.

However, introductions to date have paid minimal attention to its contribution to the travel memoir form. Rather, the book is described as the first autobiography written by a woman of mixed-race in Britain or, incorrectly, the first by a black woman. In fact, the first autobiography by a black woman was by a freed slave in 1831, *The History of Mary Prince, a West Indian Slave, Related by Herself.*

The anonymous reviewer in *The Critic* (cited in Chapter 3, p 96) was highly positive about the book, although he suggested that Seacole, a 'jolly old soul,' had 'evidently not written a line of it,' but since she 'furnished the materials to the editor,' that was enough. The book was 'pleasant and readable — aye, and as instructive a little volume as a man need take up for a couple of hours' amusement.' He gave numerous extracts and a thorough synopsis of the events of her life, with fewer errors than is typical today. There is no suggestion that she won medals or risked her life and her services are called 'suttling,' her goods sold not to soldiers, but to officers, who called her 'mother.' She was praised for her kindness, having a good word for everyone, being 'a skillful nurse and doctress' and telling her stories with a 'charming air of simplicity and good faith' (322). The reviewer did not think well of Russell's preface to the book, but endorsed his call for funds to assist her (321). The next review, which was heavy on extracts, was complimentary both to Seacole and Russell. She had 'a warm heart and a courageous disposition,' which she turned to good account. The events of her life were 'strange and in some instances startling' and she told her story 'amusingly.' But there is no mention of medals or heroism on the battlefield and instead of her 'saving thousands,' as is so often said now, she merely 'earned the good will and gratitude of hundreds.'[1]

Another lengthy, sympathetic review, also with extracts, appeared soon after in *The Lady's Newspaper*. It noted that a fund had been started by a 'very influential body of noblemen and gentlemen' and hoped that the sale of the book would help Seacole 'to repair her shattered fortune.'[2] The periodical had earlier given sympathetic coverage to her bankruptcy (29 November 1856).

The revival of interest in Seacole in the late twentieth century led to the production of new editions: five major ones with editorial introductions between 1984 and 2009 (listed in the References), plus numerous others in various formats: hard cover, paperback, e-books and large print. The book has long been in the public domain, which makes new editions easy to produce and they continue to appear. The five introductions mentioned above all have obvious factual errors. In length, they range from three pages (Cadogan) to over thirty-five pages (both the Oxford and Penguin editions). The Oxford edition has the fewest errors and generally provides the best coverage of the issues. The edition by Washington is by far the most inaccurate.

Excerpts from *Wonderful Adventures* follow, beginning with her travels in Panama and life in Jamaica.

---

[1] 'Literature,' review of Wonderful Adventures of Mrs Seacole in Many Lands, *Illustrated London News* 31,870 (25 July 1857):102.

[2] Review, *The Lady's Newspaper* 1 August 1857 p 70.

Arrival at her brother's hotel in Panama, Chapter 3, 217-21

The sympathizing reader...can fancy that I was looking forward with no little pleasurable anticipation to reaching my brother's cheerful home at Cruces. After the long night spent on board the wretched boat in my stiff, clayey, dress, and the hours of fasting, the warmth and good cheer of the Independent Hotel could not fail to be acceptable.

My brother met me on the rickety wharf with the kindest welcome in his face, although he did not attempt to conceal a smile at my forlorn appearance....On our way, he rather damped my hopes by expressing his fears that he should be unable to provide his sister with the accommodation he could wish. For you see, he said, the crowd from Panama has just come in, meeting your crowd from Navy Bay, and I should not be at all surprised if very many of them have no better bed than the store floors. But, despite this warning, I was miserably unprepared for the reception that awaited me....

Picture to yourself, sympathizing reader, a long, low hut, built of rough, unhewn, unplaned logs, filled up with mud and split bamboo, a long, sloping roof and a large verandah, already full of visitors....At the entrance sat a black man taking toll of the comers-in, giving them in exchange for coin or gold dust (he had a rusty pair of scales to weigh the latter) a dirty ticket, which guaranteed them supper, a night's lodging and breakfast. I saw all this very quickly, and turned round upon my brother in angry despair....

At last he made room for me in a corner of the crowded bar, set before me some food and left me to watch the strange life I had come to...

As the evening wore on, the shouting and quarrelling at the doorway in Yankee twang increased momentarily, while some seated themselves at the table, and hammering upon it with the handles of their knives, hallooed out to the excited nigger cooks to make haste with the slapjack. Amidst all this confusion, my brother was quietly selling shirts, boots, trousers, etc., to the travellers, while above all the din could be heard the screaming voices of his touters without, drawing attention to the good cheer of the Independent Hotel....

At last the table was nearly filled with a motley assemblage of men and women, and the slapjack, hot and steaming, was carried in by the black cooks.

Cholera in Panama, Chapter 4, 26–32

It was scarcely surprising that the cholera should spread rapidly, for fear is its powerful auxiliary, and the Cruces people bowed down before the plague in slavish despair. The Americans and other foreigners in the place showed a brave front, but the natives, constitutionally cowardly, made not the feeblest show of resistance. Beyond filling the poor church, and making the priests bring out into the streets figures of tawdry dirty saints, supposed to possess some miraculous influence which they never exerted, before which they prostrated themselves, invoking their aid with passionate prayers and cries, they did nothing. Very likely the saints would have got the credit for helping them if they had helped themselves, but the poor cowards never stirred a finger to clean out their close, reeking, huts, or rid the damp streets of the rotting accumulation of months. I think their chief reliance was on 'the yellow woman from Jamaica with the cholera medicine.' Nor was this surprising, for the Spanish doctor who was sent for from Panama became nervous and frightened at the horrors around him, and the people soon saw that he was not familiar with the terrible disease...and preferred trusting to one who was.

It must be understood that many of those who could afford to pay for my services did so handsomely, but the great majority of my patients had nothing better to give their doctress than thanks....

It was late in the evening when the largest mule owner in Cruces came to me and implored me to accompany him to his kraal, a short distance from the town, where he said some of his men were dying....

The groans of the sufferers and the anxiety and fear of their comrades were so painful to hear and witness....The mule owner was so frightened that he did not hesitate to obey orders, and, by my directions, doors and shutters were thrown open, fires were lighted and every effort made to ventilate the place, and then, with the aid of the frightened women, I applied myself to my poor patients. Two were beyond my skill. Death alone could give them relief. The others I could help....

I found the worst cases sinking fast, one of the others had relapsed, while fear had paralysed the efforts of the rest. At last I restored some order and, with the help of the bravest of the women, fixed up rude screens around the dying men. But no screens could shut out from the others their awful groans and cries for the aid that no mortal power could give them. So the long night passed away, first a deathlike stillness behind one screen, and then a sudden silence behind the other, showing that the fierce battle with death was over....

Meanwhile, I sat before the flickering fire with my last patient in my lap, a poor, little, brown-faced orphan infant, scarce a year old, was dying in my arms, and I was powerless to save it. It may seem strange, but it is a fact that I thought more of that little child than I did of the men who were struggling for their lives, and prayed very earnestly and solemnly to God to spare it. But it did not please him to grant my prayer, and towards morning the wee spirit left this sinful world for the home above it had so lately left, and what was mortal of the little infant lay dead in my arms.

Then it was that I began to think...that, if it were possible to take this little child and examine it, I should learn more of the terrible disease which was sparing neither young nor old, and should know better how to do battle with it....I followed the man who had taken the dead child away to bury it, and bribed him to carry it by an unfrequented path down to the riverside....Having persuaded him thus much, it was not difficult, with the help of silver arguments, to convince him that it would be for the general benefit and his own if I could learn from this poor little thing the secret inner workings of our common foe, and ultimately he stayed by me and aided me in my first and last *postmortem* examination. It seems a strange deed to accomplish, and I am sure I could not wield the scalpel or the substitute I then used now, but at that time the excitement had strung my mind up to a high pitch of courage and determination....

I need not linger on this scene, nor give the readers the results of my operation, although novel to me, and decidedly useful, they were what every medical man well knows. We buried the poor little body beneath a piece of luxuriant turf, and stole back into Cruces like guilty things. But the knowledge I had obtained thus strangely was very valuable to me and was soon put into practice.

I would fain give [readers] some idea of my treatment of this terrible disease. I have no doubt that at first I made some lamentable blunders and, may be, lost patients which, a little later, I could have saved. I know I came across, the other day, some notes of cholera medicines which made me shudder, and I dare say they have been used in their turn and found wanting.

The simplest remedies were perhaps the best: mustard plasters and emetics and calomel, the mercury applied externally where the veins were nearest the surface, were my usual resources. Opium I rather dreaded, as its effect is to incapacitate the system from making any exertion, and it lulls the patient into a sleep which is often the sleep of death.

When my patients felt thirsty, I would give them water in which cinnamon had been boiled. One stubborn attack succumbed to an additional dose of ten grains of sugar of lead, mixed in a pint of water, given in doses of a tablespoonful every quarter of an hour. Another patient, a girl, I rubbed over with warm oil, camphor and spirits of wine. Above all, I never neglected to apply mustard poultices to the stomach, spine and neck, and particularly to keep my patient warm about the region of the heart....

One great conclusion which my practice in cholera cases enabled me to come to was the old one, that few constitutions permitted the use of exactly similar remedies, and that the course of treatment which saved one man would, if persisted in, have very likely killed his brother.

American Independence Day in Panama, Chapter 6, 46–48

The most important social meeting took place on the anniversary of the Declaration of American Independence, at my brother's hotel, where a score of zealous Americans dined most heartily — as they never fail to do, and, as it was an especial occasion, drank champagne....After the usual patriotic toasts had been duly honoured, they proposed 'the ladies,' with an especial reference to myself, in a speech which I thought worth noting down at the time.

The spokesman was a thin, sallow looking American, with a pompous and yet rapid delivery.... 'Well, gentlemen, I expect you all support me in a drinking of this toast that I do — Aunty Seacole, gentlemen — I give you Aunty Seacole. We can't do less for her after what she's done for us, when the cholera was among us...not many months ago. So I say, God bless the best yaller woman he ever made — from Jamaica, gentlemen....I expect there are only two things we're vexed for and the first is that she ain't one of us — a citizen of the great United States — and the other thing is...that Providence made her a yaller woman. I calculate, gentlemen, you're all as vexed as I am that she's not wholly white...and I guess if we could bleach her by any means we would and thus make her as acceptable in any company as she deserves to be. Gentlemen, I give you Aunty Seacole!'...

[Seacole:] 'Gentlemen, I return you my best thanks for your kindness in drinking my health....But I must say that I don't altogether appreciate your friend's kind wishes with respect to my complexion. If it had been as dark as any nigger's, I should have been just as happy and as useful, and as much respected by those whose respect I value, and as to his offer of bleaching me, I should, even if it were practicable, decline it without any thanks. As to the society which the process might gain me admission into, all I can say is that, judging from the specimens I have met with here and elsewhere, I don't think that I shall lose much by being excluded from it. So, gentlemen, I drink to you and the general reformation of American manners.'

A yellow fever epidemic in Jamaica, Chapter 7, 59–61, 63

I stayed in Jamaica eight months out of the year 1853, still remembered in the island for its suffering and gloom....My house was full of sufferers — officers, their wives and children. Very often they were borne in from the ships in the harbour, sometimes in a dying state, sometimes — after long and distressing struggles with the grim foe — to recover. Habituated as I had become with death in its most harrowing forms, I found these scenes more difficult to bear than any I had previously borne a part in....It was a terrible thing to see young people in the youth and bloom of life suddenly stricken down, not in battle with an enemy that threatened their country, but in vain contest with a climate that refused to adopt them....

I cannot trace *all* the peace and resignation which I have witnessed on many death beds to temperament alone, although I believe it has much more to do with them than many teachers will allow. I have stood by receiving the last blessings of Christians, and closing the eyes of those who had nothing to trust to but the mercy of a God who will be far more merciful to us than we are to one another....

After this, I was sent for by the medical authorities to provide nurses for the sick at Up-Park Camp, about a mile from Kingston, and, leaving some nurses and my sister at home, I went there and did my best, but it was very little we could do to mitigate the severity of the epidemic.

Gold prospecting in Escribanos, Panama 66–72

Carlos Alexander, the alcide [strong man] of Escribanos, had made a good thing out of the gold mania. The mine had belonged to him, had been sold at a fine price and, passing through several hands, had at last come into possession of the company who were now working it, its former owner settling down as ruler over the little community of two hundred souls....He was a black man, was fond of talking of his early life in slavery and how he had escaped, and possessed no ordinary intellect. He possessed, also, a house, which in England a well-bred hound would not have accepted as a kennel, a white wife and a pretty daughter with a whitey-brown complexion and a pleasant name, Juliana....

I did not stay long at Escribanos on my first visit as the alcide's guest, but, having made arrangements for a longer sojourn, I went back to Navy Bay, where I laid in a good stock of the stores I should have most use for, and returned to Escribanos in safety. I remained there some months, pleased with the novelty of the life and busy with schemes for seeking for or, as the gold diggers call it, prospecting for other mines....

In consequence of the difficulty of communication with Navy Bay, our fare was of the simplest at Escribanos. It consisted mainly of salt meat, rice and roasted Indian corn. The native fare was not tempting, and some of their delicacies were absolutely disgusting. With what pleasure, for instance, could one foreign to their tastes and habits dine off a roasted monkey, whose grilled head bore a strong resemblance to a negro baby's? And yet the Indians used to bring them to us for sale, strung on a stick. They were worse still stewed in soup, when it was positively frightful to dip your ladle in unsuspectingly, and bring up what closely resembled a brown baby's limb. I got on better with the parrots, and could agree with the 'senorita, buono buono' with which the natives recommended them, and yet their flesh, what little there was of it, was very coarse and hard. Nor did I always refuse to concede praise to a squirrel, if well cooked. But, although the flesh of the iguana — another favourite dish — was white and tender as any chicken, I never could stomach it....

The tropical scenery was very grand, but I am afraid I only marked what was most curious in it — at least, that is, foremost in my memory now. I know I wondered much what motive Nature could have had in twisting the roots and branches of the trees into such strange, fantastic, contortions....

Soon after this, I left Escribanos and, stopping but a short time at Navy Bay, came on direct to England. I had claims on a mining company which are still unsatisfied. I had to look after my share in the Palmilla Mine speculation....

I found something to admire in the people of New Granada, but not much, and I found very much more to condemn most unequivocally. Whatever was of any worth in their institutions, such as their comparative freedom, religious toleration, etc., was owing mainly to the negroes who had sought the protection of the republic. I found the Spanish Indians treacherous, passionate and indolent, with no higher aim or object but simply to enjoy the present after their own torpid, useless, fashion. Like most fallen nations, they are very conservative in their habits and principles, while the blacks are enterprising and in their opinions incline not unnaturally to democracy.

Arrival and early weeks in the Crimea, 96–98, 100–01

I remained six weeks in Balaclava, spending my days on shore and my nights on board ship. Over our stores, stacked on the shore, a few sheets of rough tarpaulin were suspended, and beneath these — my sole protection against the Crimean rain and wind — I spent some portion of each day, receiving visitors and selling stores.

But my chief occupation, and one with which I never allowed any business to interfere, was helping the doctors to transfer the sick and wounded from the mules and ambulances into the transports that had to carry them to the hospitals of Scutari and Buyukdere [northern Constantinople]....

My acquaintance with it [the wharf] began very shortly after I had reached Balaclava. The very first day that I approached the wharf, a party of sick and wounded had just arrived. Here was work for me, I felt sure. With so many patients, the doctors must be glad of all the hands they could get....I do not think that the surgeons noticed me at first, although, as this was my introduction to Balaclava, I had not neglected my personal appearance and wore my favourite yellow dress and blue bonnet with the red ribbons, but I noticed one coming to me, who, I think, would have laughed very merrily had it not been for the poor fellow at my feet. As it was, he came forward and shook hands very kindly, saying, 'How do you do, ma'am? Much obliged to you for looking after my poor fellow, very glad to see you here.' And glad they always were, the kind-hearted doctors, to let me help them look after the sick and wounded sufferers brought to that fearful wharf.

But it must not be supposed that we had no cheerful scenes upon the sick wharf. Sometimes a light-hearted fellow — generally a sailor — would forget his pain and do his best to keep the rest in good spirits. Once I heard my name eagerly pronounced, and, turning round, recognized a sailor whom I remembered as one of the crew of the *Alarm* stationed at Kingston a few years back.

'Why, as I live, if this ain't Aunty Seacole of Jamaica! Shiver all that's left of my poor timbers,' and I saw that the left leg was gone — 'if this ain't a rum go, mates!'

'Ah! my man, I'm sorry to see you in this sad plight.'

'Never fear for me, Aunty Seacole, I'll make the best of the leg the Rooshians have left me. I'll get at them soon again, never fear....'

'You bear your troubles well, my son.'

'Eh! do I, Aunty?' and he seemed surprised. 'Why, look ye, when I've seen so many pretty fellows knocked off the ship's roll altogether, don't you think I ought to be thankful if I can answer the bo'swain's call anyhow?'

And this was the sailors' philosophy always, and this brave fellow, after he had sipped some lemonade and laid down, when he heard the men groaning, raised his head and comforted them in the same strain again, and, it may seem strange, but it quieted them.

I used to make sponge cakes on board the *Medora*, with eggs brought from Constantinople. Only the other day, Captain S., who had charge of the *Medora*, reminded me of them. These, with some lemonade, were all the doctors would allow me to give to the wounded. They all liked the cake, poor fellows, better than anything else, perhaps because it tasted of 'home.'

Thieves, Chapter 11, 104–06

The thievery in this little out-of-the way port was something marvellous, and the skill and ingenuity of the operators would have reflected credit upon the *élite* of their profession practising in the most civilized city of Europe. Nor was the thievery confined altogether to the professionals who had crowded to this scene of action from the cities and islands of the Mediterranean. They robbed us, the Turks, and one another....

In this predatory warfare, as in more honourable service, the Zouaves [French Algerians] particularly distinguished themselves. These undoubtedly gallant little fellows, always restless for action of some sort, would, when the luxury of a brush with the Russians was occasionally denied them, come down to Balaclava in search of opportunities of waging war against society at large. Their complete and utter absence of conscientious scruples as to the rights of property was most amusing.

To see a Zouave gravely cheat a Turk, or trip up a Greek street merchant or Maltese fruit seller, and scud away with the spoil, cleverly stowed in his roomy red pantaloons, was an operation for its coolness, expedition and perfectness well worth seeing. And, to a great extent, they escaped scatheless, for the English provost marshal's department was rather chary of interfering with the eccentricities of our gallant allies, while, if the French had taken close cognizance of the Zouaves' amusements out of school, one half of the regiments would have been always engaged punishing the other half.

The poor Turk! It is lamentable to think how he was robbed, abused and bullied by his friends. Why didn't he show a little pluck?

Meeting Omar Pasha, Chapter 11, 110–11

My visit to the Turkish pasha laid the foundation of a lasting friendship. He soon found his way to Spring Hill, and before long became one of my best customers and most frequent visitors. It was astonishing to note how completely, now that he was in the land of the Giaours [infidels], he adapted himself to the tastes and habits of the infidels. Like a Scotch Presbyterian on the Continent for a holiday, he threw aside all the prejudices of his education and drank bottled beer, sherry and champagne, with an appreciation of their qualities that no thirsty-souled Christian could have expressed more gratefully. He was very affable with us all, and would sometimes keep Jew Johnny away from his work for hours, chatting with us or the English officers who would lounge into our as yet unfinished store. Sometimes he would come down to breakfast and spend the greater part of the day at Spring Hill....

The pasha's great ambition was to be familiar with the English language, and at last nothing would do but he would take lessons of me. So he would come down and, sitting in my store, with a Turk or so at his feet to attend to his most important pipe, by inserting little red hot pieces of charcoal at intervals, would try hard to sow a few English sentences in his treacherous memory. He never got beyond half a dozen, and I think if we had continued in the relation of pupil and mistress until now, the number would not have been increased greatly. 'Madame Seacole,' 'Gentlemen, good morning,' and 'More champagne,' with each syllable much dwelt upon, were his favourite sentences. It was capital fun to hear him....

Very frequently he would compliment me by ordering his band down to Spring Hill for my amusement. They played excellently well, and I used to think that I preferred their music to that of the French and English regimental bands. I laughed heartily one day when, in compliance with the kind-hearted Anglo-Turkish pasha's orders, they came out with a grand new tune, in which I with difficulty recognized a very distant resemblance to 'God Save the Queen.'

Altogether he was a capital neighbour, and gave such strict orders to his men to respect our property that we rarely lost anything. On the whole, the Turks were the most honest of the nations there (I except the English and the Sardinians) and the most tractable. But the Greeks hated them, and showed their hate in every way.

Food and catering, Chapter 11, 141, 145, 150–51

I had a reputation for my sponge cakes that any pastry cook in London...might have been proud of. The officers, full of fun and high spirits, used to crowd into the little kitchen, and, despite all my remonstrances, which were not always confined to words, for they made me frantic sometimes, and an iron spoon is a tempting weapon, would carry off the tarts hot from the oven, while the good-for-nothing black cooks, instead of lending me their aid, would stand by and laugh with all their teeth. And when the hot season commenced, the crowds that came to the British Hotel for my claret and cider cups, and other cooling summer drinks, were very complimentary in their expressions of appreciation of my skill.

Until evening, the store would be filled with customers wanting stores, dinners and luncheons, loungers and idlers seeking conversation and amusement, and at eight o'clock the curtain descended on that day's labour and I could sit down and eat at leisure. It was no easy thing to clear the store, canteen and yards, but we determined upon adhering to the rule that nothing should be sold after that hour, and succeeded. Anyone who came after that time came simply as a friend.

During May, and while preparations were being made for the third great bombardment of the ill-fated city, summer broke beautifully, and the weather, chequered occasionally by fitful intervals of cold and rain, made us all cheerful....It was a period of relaxation and they all enjoyed it. Amusement was the order of the day. Races, dog hunts, cricket matches and dinner parties were eagerly indulged in, and in all I could be of use to provide the good cheer which was so essential a part of these entertainments, and when the warm weather came in all its intensity, and I took to manufacturing cooling beverages for my friends and customers, my store was always full....

In anticipation of the hot weather, I had laid in a large stock of raspberry vinegar which, properly managed, helps to make a pleasant drink, and there was a great demand for sangaree [sangria], claret and cider cups, the cups being battered pewter pots. Would you like, reader, to know my recipe for the favourite claret cup? It is simple enough: claret, water, lemon peel, sugar, nutmeg and ice — yes, ice — but not often and not for long, for the eager officers soon made an end of it.

Sometimes there were dinner parties at Spring Hill....At one of the earliest, when the *Times* correspondent was to be present, I rode down to Kadikoi, bought some calico and cut it up into table napkins. They all laughed very heartily, and thought perhaps of a few weeks previously, when every available piece of linen in the camp would have been snapped up for pocket handkerchiefs.

Battles and death, Chapter 15, 147–48, 152, 155–59

My first experience of battle was pleasant enough. Before we had been long at Spring Hill, Omar Pasha got something for his Turks to do, and one fine morning they were marched away towards the Russian outposts on the road to Baidar. I accompanied them on horseback, and enjoyed the sight amazingly. English and French cavalry preceded the Turkish infantry over the plain, yet full of memorials of the terrible Light Cavalry charge a few months before [in the Battle of Balaclava] and, while one detachment of the Turks made a reconnaissance to the right of the Tchernaya [River], another pushed their way up the hill, towards Kamara, driving in the Russian outposts after what seemed but a slight resistance. It was very pretty to see them advance and to watch how every now and then little clouds of white smoke puffed up from behind bushes and the crests of hills, and were answered by similar puffs from the long line of busy skirmishers that preceded the main body. This was my first experience of actual battle.

The deaths in the trenches touched me deeply....It was very usual, when a young officer was ordered into the trenches, for him to ride down to Spring Hill to dine, or obtain something more than his ordinary fare to brighten his weary hours in those fearful ditches. They seldom failed on these occasions to shake me by the hand at parting, and sometimes would say, 'You see, Mrs Seacole, I can't say good-bye to the dear ones at home, so I'll bid you good-bye for them. Perhaps you'll see them some day, and, if the Russians should knock me over, Mother, just tell them I thought of them all, will you?' And although all this might be said in a light-hearted manner, it was rather solemn.

In the first week of June, the third bombardment of Sebastopol opened, and the Spring Hill visitors had plenty to talk about....Somehow or other, important secrets oozed out in various parts of the camp which the Russians would have given much to know, and one of these places was the British Hotel. Some such whispers were afloat on the evening of Sunday the 17th of June....I never remember feeling more excited or more restless than upon that day, and no sooner had night fairly closed in upon us than, instead of making preparations for bed...[I started] off for a long walk to Cathcart's Hill, three miles and a half away. I stayed there until past midnight, but when I returned home there was no rest for me, for I had found out that, in the stillness of the night, many regiments were marching down to the trenches, and that the dawn of day would be the signal that should let them loose upon the Russians. The few hours still left before daybreak were made the most of at Spring Hill.

We were all busily occupied in cutting bread and cheese and sandwiches, packing up fowls, tongues and ham, wine and spirits, while I carefully filled the large bag which I always carried into the field slung across my shoulder, with lint, bandages, needles, thread and medicines and, soon after daybreak, everything was ready packed upon two mules, in charge of my steadiest lad, and I leading the way on horseback, the little cavalcade left...before the sun of the fatal 18th of June had been many hours old....

I reached Cathcart's Hill crowded with non-combatants and, leaving there the mules, loaded myself with what provisions I could carry, and — it was a work of no little difficulty and danger — succeeded in reaching the reserves of Sir Henry Barnard's division, which was to have stormed something, I forget what, but when they found the attack upon the Redan was a failure, very wisely abstained. Here I found plenty of officers who soon relieved me of my refreshments and some wounded men who found the contents of my bag very useful.

At length I made my way to the Woronozoff Road, where the temporary hospital had been erected, and there I found the doctors hard enough at work, and hastened to help them as best I could. I bound up the wounds and ministered to the wants of a good many, and stayed there some considerable time....

While at the hospital I was chiefly of use looking after those, who, either from lack of hands or because their hurts were less serious, had to wait, pained and weary, until the kind-hearted doctors, who however *looked* more like murderers — could attend to them....

After this, first washing my hands in some sherry from lack of water, I went back to Cathcart's Hill, where I found my horse, and heard that the good-for-nothing lad, either frightened or tired of waiting, had gone away with the mules. I had to ride three miles after him, and then the only satisfaction I had arose from laying my horse whip about his shoulders. After that, working my way round, how I can scarcely tell, I got to the extreme left attack, where General Eyre's division had been hotly engaged all day and had suffered severely. I left my horse in charge of some men, and, with no little difficulty and at no little risk, crept down to where some wounded men lay, with whom I left refreshments. And then — it was growing late — I started for Spring Hill, where I heard all about the events of the luckless day from those who had seen them from posts of safety....

That evening of the 18th of June was a sad one, and the news that came in of those that had fallen were most heartrending. Both the leaders who fell so gloriously before the Redan had been very good to the mistress of Spring Hill [Colonel Yea and Sir John Campbell].

The last bombardment and fall of Sebastopol, Chapter 17, 168–70, 172–74, 176–77

I spent much of my time on Cathcart's Hill watching, with a curiosity and excitement which became intense, the progress of the terrible bombardment. Now and then a shell would fall among the crowd of on-lookers which covered the hill, but it never disturbed us, so keen and feverish and so deadened to danger had the excitement and expectation made us.

In the midst of the bombardment took place the important ceremony of distributing the Order of the Bath [27 August 1855] to those selected for that honour. I contrived to witness this ceremony very pleasantly, and although it cost me a day, I considered that I had fairly earned the pleasure. I was anxious to have some personal share in the affair, so I made and forwarded to headquarters a cake...and which I adorned gaily with banners, flags, etc. I received great kindness from the officials at the ceremony and from the officers — some of rank — who recognized me; indeed I held quite a little *levée* around my chair....

The firing began at early dawn and was fearful. Sleep was impossible, so I arose and set out for my old station on Cathcart's Hill. And here, with refreshments for the anxious lookers-on, I spent most of my time, right glad of any excuse to witness the last scene of the siege. It was from this spot that I saw fire after fire break out in Sebastopol, and watched all night the beautiful yet terrible effect of a great ship blazing in the harbour, and lighting up the adjoining country for miles....

The morning of the memorable 8th of September broke cold and wintry. The same little bird which had let me into so many secrets also gave me a hint of what this day was pregnant with, and very early in the morning I was on horseback, with my bandages and refreshments, ready to repeat the work of the 18th of June last....So, early in the day I was in my old spot.

It was noon before the cannonading suddenly ceased, and we saw, with a strange feeling of excitement, the French tumble out of their advanced trenches and roll into the Malakhoff like a human flood....And, before this, our men had made their attack and the fearful assault of the Redan was going on and failing. But I was soon too busy to see much, for the wounded were borne in even in greater numbers than at the last assault....I saw many officers of the 97th wounded, and as far as possible I reserved my attentions for my old regiment, known so well in my native island.

I remained on Cathcart's Hill far into the night, and watched the city blazing beneath us, awestruck at the terrible sight, until the bitter wind found its way through my thin clothing and chilled me to the bone, and not till then did I leave for Spring Hill. I had little sleep that night. The night was made a ruddy lurid day with the glare of the blazing town, while every now and then came reports which shook the earth to its centre....In the night, covered by the burning city, Sebastopol was left a heap of ruins to its victors and, before noon on the following day, none but dead and dying Russians were in the south side of the once famous and beautiful...city....

The news of the evacuation of Sebastopol soon carried away all traces of yesterday's fatigue. For weeks past I had been offering bets to everyone that I would not only be the first woman to enter Sebastopol from the English lines, but that I would be the first to carry refreshments into the fallen city. And now the time I had longed for had come. I borrowed some mules from the Land Transport Corps — mine were knocked up by yesterday's work — and, loading them with good things, started off with my partner and some other friends early on that memorable Sunday morning for Cathcart's Hill....

So many attached themselves to my staff, becoming for the nonce my attendants, that I had some difficulty at starting....

I can give you no very clear description of its condition on that Sunday morning a year and a half ago. Many parts of it were still blazing furiously — explosions were taking place in all directions — every step had a score of dangers, and yet curiosity and excitement carried us on and on. I was often stopped to give refreshments to officers and men who had been fasting for hours. Some, on the other hand, had found their way to Russian cellars, and one body of men were most ingloriously drunk and playing the wildest pranks. They were dancing, yelling and singing — some of them with Russian women's dresses fastened round their waists, and old bonnets stuck upon their heads.

I was offered many trophies. All plunder was stopped by the sentries and confiscated, so that the soldiers could afford to be liberal. By one I was offered a great velvet sofa; another pressed a huge armchair, which had graced some Sebastopol study, upon me; while a third begged my acceptance of a portion of a grand piano. What I did carry away was very unimportant: a gaily decorated altar candle, studded with gold and silver stars, which the present commander-in-chief condescended to accept as a Sebastopol memorial, an old cracked China teapot...a cracked bell, which had run many to prayers during the siege, and which I bore away on my saddle, and a parasol, given me by a drunken soldier.

On the following day, I again entered Sebastopol and saw still more of its horrors. But I have refrained from describing so many scenes of woe that I am loath to dwell much on these. The very recollection of that woeful hospital, where thousands of dead and dying had been left by the retreating Russians, is enough to unnerve the strongest and sicken the most experienced. I would give much if I had never seen that harrowing sight.... I made my way into the Redan also, although every step was dangerous, and took from it some brown bread, which seemed to have been left in the oven by the baker when he fled.

Before many days were passed, some French women opened houses in Sebastopol, but in that quarter of the town held by the English the prospect was not sufficiently tempting for me to follow their example, and so I saw out the remainder of the campaign from my old quarters at Spring Hill.

After the fall of Sebastopol, Chapter 18, 177–79

Well, the great work was accomplished — Sebastopol was taken. The Russians had retired sullenly to their stronghold on the north side of the harbour, from which, every now and then, they sent a few vain shot and shell, which sent the amateurs in the streets of Sebastopol scampering, but gave the experienced no concern....

All who were before Sebastopol will long remember the beautiful autumn which succeeded to so eventful a summer, and ushered in so pleasantly the second winter of the campaign. It was appreciated as only those who earn the right to enjoyment can enjoy relaxation. The camp was full of visitors of every rank. They thronged the streets of Sebastopol, sketching its ruins and setting up photographic apparatus, in contemptuous indifference of the shot with which the Russians generally favoured every conspicuous group.

Pleasure was hunted keenly. Cricket matches, picnics, dinner parties, races, theatricals, all found their admirers. My restaurant was always full, and once more merry laughter was heard, and many a dinner party was held beneath the iron roof....Several were given in compliment to our allies, and many distinguished Frenchmen have tested my powers of cooking. You might have seen at one party some of their most famous officers. At once were present a prince of the imperial family of France, the duc de Rouchefoucault, and a certain corporal in the French service, who was perhaps the best known man in the whole army, the Viscount Talon. They expressed themselves highly gratified at the *carte*, and perhaps were not a little surprised as course after course made its appearance, and soup and fish succeeded turkeys, saddle of mutton, fowls, ham, tongue, curry, pastry of many sorts, custards, jelly, blancmange and olives. I took a peculiar pride in doing my best when they were present, for I knew a little of the secrets of the French commissariat....

I wonder if the system of secrecy which has so long kept veiled the sufferings of the French Army before Sebastopol will ever yield to truth. I used to guess something of those sufferings when I saw, even after the fall of Sebastopol, half-starved French soldiers prowling about my store, taking eagerly even what the Turks rejected as unfit for human food, and no one could accuse *them* of squeamishness, I cannot but believe that in some desks or bureaux the notes or diaries which shall one day be given to the world, and when this happens the terrible distresses of the English Army will pall before the unheard of sufferings of the French. It is true that they carried from Sebastopol the lion's share of glory. My belief is that they deserved it, having borne by far a larger proportion of suffering.

Christmas 1855, 185–87

Christmas came and with it pleasant memories of home and of home comforts....I wonder if the people of other countries are as fond of carrying with them everywhere their home habits as the English. I think not. I think there was something purely and essentially English in the determination of the camp to spend the Christmas Day of 1855 after the good old 'home' fashion. It showed itself weeks before the eventful day, in the dinner parties which were got up, in the orders sent to England — in the supplies which came out, and in the many applications made to the hostess...for plum puddings and mince pies....

For three week previous to Christmas Day, my time was fully occupied in making preparations for it. Pages of my books are filled with orders for plum puddings and mince pies, beside which I sold an immense quantity of raw material to those who were too far off to send down for the manufactured article on Christmas Day....

From an early hour in the morning until long after the night had set in, were I and my cooks busy endeavouring to supply the great demand for Christmas fare. We had considerable difficulty in keeping our engagements, but by substituting mince pies for plum puddings, in a few cases, we succeeded. The scene in the crowded store and even in the little overheated kitchen, with the officers' servants who came in for their masters' dinners, cannot well be described. Some were impatient themselves, others dreaded their masters' impatience as the appointed dinner hour passed by....Angry cries for the major's plum pudding, which was to have been ready an hour ago, alternated with an entreaty that I should cook the captain's mince pies to a turn....

I did not get my dinner until eight o'clock, and then I dined in peace off a fine wild turkey or bustard, shot for me on the marshes by the Tchernaya. It weighed twenty two pounds and, although somewhat coarse in colour, had a capital flavour.

Upon New Year's Day, I had another large cooking of plum puddings and mince pies, this time upon my own account. I took them to the hospital of the Land Transport Corps, to remind the patients of the home comforts they longed so much for.

227

Chapter 7

What next?

Seacole without the myths

What's left when the exaggerations and misrepresentations are removed from Seacole's biography? A lot. The life Seacole made for herself was full of adventures and her memoir recounting them is a fine book. She travelled independently when few women did. She faced adversities and surmounted them. She was a businesswoman, mainly successful. She pursued her avocation as 'doctress' or herbalist to the satisfaction of many.

She faced racial prejudice, especially by Southern Americans, and dealt with it admirably. She had confidence in her own worth and insisted on the equality of all people, regardless of race. Her response to the American man who toasted her and wished her skin could be bleached was splendid.

As well as running her business, Seacole gave time and effort to voluntary service. She provided her remedies without charge to those who could not pay for them. She gave comfort and consolation when she could not hope to cure. During the Crimean War, she made extra food in her kitchen for sick soldiers — rice pudding was a favourite for her officer customers and a large pan on occasion went to the Land Transport Corps Hospital. This is all commendable, if short of the claims made about her.

During the war, Seacole made friends with her customers. She provided good food, if expensive, in a convivial atmosphere. Nightingale herself remarked on her kindness, especially to officers. When her business failed, her customers rallied round to support her. All the above is based on sound information, not myth. The claims of her being a pioneer nurse, nurse practitioner, pharmacist or physician belong to the 'fake history.'

Seacole adapted easily to British life, it seems, having imbibed the values and ways of the empire in Jamaica and witnessed scenes that showed American values and ways at their worst. Jamaicans were encouraged to identify with the mother country and she did, with enthusiasm. She distanced herself from her African heritage and used racist language for blacks, not considering herself one. As a Jamaican, she had no interest in the Crimean War, but her loyalty to the British Army and British Empire motivated her to go to it. She was an early successful immigrant to Britain, adapted to its customs and was appreciated for what she brought to the country.

Seacole enjoyed celebrity status in the immediate post-war period. She got frequent press coverage merely for appearing at an event and press descriptions of her were routinely favourable. She even had a horse named after her! She was not 'the first black woman to make her mark in British public life,' but she was the first mixed-race person to have done so.

Her supporters seldom mention an interesting aspect of her life, her late conversion to Roman Catholicism. Nothing is known as to when and why, but, in the circumstances, conversion could only mean serious conviction. There was nothing to gain in Protestant England by joining the politically and socially disadvantaged Roman Catholics.

The promotion of Mary Seacole as a 'black Briton' has obviously met a deeply felt need for more representative heroes and heroines, especially in the beleaguered National Health Service. But what kind? My surmise is that it will not be long before a whistle blower complains about the fake historical 'facts.' Perhaps a historian will do the deed, or a nurse or doctor, who insists on historical veracity for their models. It is only a question of time before black Britons feel patronized by the false claims made for Seacole apparently on their behalf. Why not the same standards of accuracy for our models and heroes as for yours? they might ask. Indeed.

The Nightingale Society continues to defend Nightingale's reputation and presses for corrections in coverage of her (and Seacole) where they appear. Reputable institutions have begun to respond, for example, the American *National Geographic*, the UK National Army Museum and the National Archives, all of which removed errors promoting the Seacole legend.

Nursing pioneers, with diversity

Nightingale never claimed to be the sole pioneer of nursing and in fact paid tribute to those ahead of her. She mentored most of the next generation of nursing leaders, many of whom have not yet been given their due. Since her time, nursing has become much more diverse and this next contingent of nurses deserves recognition. A number of non-white nurses, some of them with Nightingale links, have made contributions worthy of celebration. Brief notes on five follow, the first herself a black 'Nightingale nurse.'

Mrs K.A. Pratt. Kofoworola Abeni Pratt (c1910–93) is a black nurse who made major contributions to the profession but has been neglected by history. She also called Nightingale her inspiration.[1] Born and brought up in Nigeria, she trained at the Nightingale School and was supported by the Nightingale Fund. She nursed at St Thomas' 1946–50, through the launching of the National Health Service in 1948. Back in Nigeria, she became the first Nigerian matron of University Hospital, Ibadan, and then the first Nigerian chief nursing officer of her country. In that capacity, she led in the 'Nigerianization' of nursing or the replacement of British nationals by Nigerians in positions of leadership.

For her accomplishments, many of them firsts, Pratt was honoured by being made a fellow of the Royal College of Nursing in 1979 and given an honorary doctorate from the University of Ife in 1981. She suffered from racial discrimination both in the UK (as an early black nurse in the NHS) and in Nigeria (when the medical service was run by white

---

[1] Justus A. Akinsanya, *An African 'Florence Nightingale': A Biography of Chief (Dr) Mrs Kofoworola Abeni Pratt.*

Britons). She is a signal link between Nightingale and her school, the National Health Service and the new diversity of nurses in health care.

(Dame) Ruth Nita Barrow (1916–95), who was born in Barbados, became a leading Caribbean nurse and social justice advocate whose work was influential throughout the region and internationally.[2] She trained at the Barbados General Hospital and the Midwifery School in Port of Spain, Trinidad, and did a diploma at the University of Toronto and another at the University of Edinburgh. She did her BSc in nursing at Columbia University, graduating in 1955.

On her return to the Caribbean, Barrow first became the principal nursing officer in Jamaica (1956), from which post she helped to shape nursing education in six Caribbean countries. She was the first matron of University College Hospital in Jamaica, the first president of the Jamaica Nurses' Association and the first Caribbean nurse appointed to the World Health Organization. Barrow was also a leader in her church and the World Council of Churches. British honours include being made a fellow of the Royal College of Nursing. She was given honorary doctorates by two Canadian universities and the University of the West Indies. In 1986 she was made a member of the Commonwealth Eminent Persons Group that visited Nelson Mandela in prison and helped set up the negotiations that ended apartheid. Her own country made her ambassador to the United Nations and then governor general of Barbados 1990–95. She was made Dame of St Andrew, of the Order of Barbados.

Dr Docia Angelina Naki Kisseih (1919-?) was the first Ghanian chief nursing officer in her country, serving from 1961 to 1974. She started her career as a midwife in 1943. In 1975, she became a lecturer in the Department of Nursing at the University of Ghana; she retired from teaching in 1981. She was president of the Ghana Registered Nurses' Association for

---

[2] Hermi Hyacinth Hewitt. *Trailblazers in Nursing Education: A Caribbean Perspective, 1946-1986.* Citation University of Manitoba.

ten years, a member of the Board of Directors of the International Council of Nurses and first vice-president of it, among many positions.

Kisseih notably led the transition to African leadership in the Ghanian nursing profession, as Pratt had in Nigeria. She was the first Ghanaian nurse to obtain a doctorate, from Boston University, where also she did her MSc in nursing. The citation on Kisseih on the Ghana Nursing Portal calls her 'a true nurse in the spirit of Florence Nightingale.'

Asoka Roy (1915–2001) was born in India, but spent much of her career as a nurse-midwife in the United States. After her initial training in New Delhi, she did a master's degree at the All-India Institute of Hygiene and Public Health in Calcutta and obtained a midwife's teaching certificate from the Royal College of Midwives in England. She later did further midwifery training in Sweden. In the course of her career, Roy delivered more than 5000 babies. During the period of partition between India and Pakistan, she made trips to war-torn villages to see her midwives to safety and to deliver babies herself. After partition, Roy became general secretary of the Trained Nurses' Association of India, the second Indian (after many Britons) to hold this post; she was the first Indian editor of its journal, *The Nursing Journal of India*. She worked also as a midwifery tutor in Britain.

In 1955, Roy emigrated to the United States, where she helped establish midwifery as a profession. She obtained a licence as a nurse-midwife in New York and became the first director of the Beth Israel Medical Center's midwifery programme. She also taught at Yale University. She was named a fellow of the American College of Nurse-Midwives. Asoka Roy's family created a 'Platinum Sponsorship' to honour her memory, the 'Koko Roy Award.'[3]

Dr Helen K. Mussallem (1915–2012), for years Canada's most influential nurse, was the first non-Briton to be made a fellow of the Royal College of Nursing. Mussallem was born in northern British Columbia, to a family of

---

[3] 'Pioneer in Nurse-Midwifery,' *New York Times* obituary 8 July 2001.

Lebanese origin. She did her nurse training at the Vancouver General Hospital 1934–37. During World War II she served as a surgical nurse in the Royal Canadian Army Medical Corps, with the rank of lieutenant. Postwar, she became director of nursing at the Vancouver General Hospital.

Mussallem was the first Canadian to earn a doctorate in nursing, at Columbia University in 1962. Her thesis was on nurse training and led to key reforms, notably the move to university education for nurses in Canada. She was executive director of the Canadian Nurses' Association 1963–81. At the CNA, Mussallem organized its significant brief, 'Putting Health Into Health Care,' which was presented to the Health Services Review of 1979, calling for a higher level of training for nurses.

Mussallem also founded the Canadian Nurses Foundation, which funds higher education for nurses. She was awarded six honorary doctorates and made a Companion of Canada, her country's highest honour. She, however, considered her greatest honour to have been given the Florence Nightingale Medal by the International Red Cross. Mussallem not only followed Nightingale as a nurse and advocate for nurse education, but as a contributor to public policy on health care.

In America, the first black nurse dates back to 1879 and the acceptance and progress of blacks in nursing has a very different history from that in the UK. There has been nothing comparable to the history faking and myth making in that history.

The ethical implications of dispensing with Nightingale as a model to replace her with Seacole seem not to have been considered by Seacole supporters. Nightingale's goal was the establishment of a respected profession which, in time, happened. Polls today show that nurses are routinely rated as trustworthy, often topping all other professions in this regard. This took decades of work, beginning in 1860 with Nightingale's insistence on assessing nursing pupils on their conduct. The categories — old-fashioned as they seem now — were 'sober, honest, truthful, punctual, quiet, trustworthy, cleanly, neat and orderly.'[4] Note the caution and repetition: honest, truthful and trustworthy are all on that list, yet are flagrantly ignored in the literature promoting Seacole over Nightingale.

There is a complication. Some young nurses and some potential nurses find inspiration in the made-up, heroic Seacole. Does the end of inspiring people justify the means — faking history? That is what the NHS Employers argue in defending their decision to name Seacole as a 'pioneer of health care,' while being unable to specify what she pioneered. Doubtless the files of NHS hospitals include many non-white nurses of merit whose life circumstances do not have to be altered to inspire. Seacole should be honoured for what she actually did, not what anybody, however worthy their objectives, says she did.

Many of the problems of nursing and health care today are matters on which Nightingale's principles are still pertinent. That is, attention to her vision and precepts would steer people in the right direction and benefit research and policy making.

Teaching on Seacole and Nightingale

According to a decision by the secretary of state for education, both Nightingale and Seacole will continue to be listed on the English National Curriculum. Drastic improvements are needed in the teaching on both, which would be most easily managed by teaching them separately. The linking of the two has resulted in limiting Nightingale's achievements to the brief period when they overlapped at the Crimean War. But her most important work took place after that, in instituting the modern profession of nursing, reforming the dreaded workhouse infirmaries, challenging the Poor Law system, making hospitals safer, pioneering statistical analysis in health care, assisting with relief measures in numerous wars after Crimea, advancing public health, famine prevention and relief in India

---

[4] In McDonald, ed., *Florence Nightingale: The Nightingale School* 149.

and along the way supporting the vote and economic rights for women. To do justice to Nightingale's significance in Britain and the world, she needs better coverage in more advanced units. Her work in statistics, research and health care policy was both significant at the time and continues to be. The lives and contributions of the two women are too different to combine teaching on them.

Coverage of Seacole to date can be faulted not only for the frequent misinformation — medals, heroism and pioneer nursing — but for detracting from her real life story and her book on it. *Wonderful Adventures* deserves coverage, although there will be challenges in dealing with the racial slurs. But these reflect the real conditions in which Seacole lived. With better resources they likely could be adequately handled. The more basic problem is the lack of reliable resources on Seacole for teaching. At the moment, published children's books on Seacole are all heavy on misinformation and myth. Websites are similarly unreliable, the BBC's the worst. Until there are adequate resources, print and electronic, there should be a moratorium on teaching Seacole in schools.

The proposal that Seacole be taught in nursing classes raises too many problems. Given that she did not leave remotely adequate case records of her remedies or outcomes, it is impossible to judge her effectiveness in any objective fashion. She made her own diagnoses and administered her own remedies, roughly based — for good and ill — on standard medical practice of the time, learned informally from doctors. She never studied medicine, nor could have.

In effect, she practised medicine without a licence, but we should be wary of seeing this as a virtue, as some of her supporters contend. She herself acknowledged 'lamentable' blunders and revisiting some of her remedies later made her shudder. Alexander Pope's 'A little knowledge is a dangerous thing' might be a better slogan than 'throw away the rule book.'

True, Nightingale insisted on a strictly limited role for nurses — no diagnosing or prescribing — while Seacole did both and with confidence. The fact remains that Seacole used harmful substances, as did many doctors of the time. Nightingale's limitation on the role of nurses was entirely reasonable given their educational qualifications at the time.

Political correctness run amuck?

The worthy object of 'political correctness' is the treatment of all people as worthy of rights and dignity, to correct historic injustices. Practically this means sensitivity to language, especially the avoidance of negative stereotypes by race, gender, religion or sexual orientation. Paying attention to these principles can help to right injustices and open up new opportunities for minorities (and women), long the victims of discrimination. The American civil rights movement, among other things, succeeded in changing public references to blacks, insisting that they be given the same honorifics and surnames as whites, instead of the usual first names, with 'Uncle' or 'Aunt' for older blacks. Such steps are only the beginning of the solution, of course, but they facilitate advocacy for better access to education, jobs and serious political roles. There is still a role for campaigns to correct past injustices.

However, the attempt to make Seacole into an exploited working-class black woman does not work. She was three-quarters white and proud of it, an owner of property and company stocks — upper middle class by any criteria. Naming her a black heroine or pioneer also raises the thorny issue of cultural appropriation. Is it right to claim an identity for someone that she herself rejected?

Meanwhile, Seacole's remarkable life and her *Wonderful Adventures* deserve to be celebrated. She did win two signal honours, in Britain by being voted the top black Briton and in Jamaica with the Order of Merit. She was an early, successful Jamaican immigrant to Britain. She combined running a business with her healing work and won recognition and even celebrity in her lifetime. It is up to the next generation of researchers to write about her work in a way that gives her due credit for her achievements and respects the historical record.

References

Editions of Seacole's Memoir in English

Seacole, Mary. *Wonderful Adventures of Mrs Seacole in Many Lands*, ed. W.J.S. London: James Blackwood 1857.
— ed. Alexander, Ziggi and Dewjee, Audrey. *Wonderful Adventures of Mrs Seacole in Many Lands*, Bristol: Falling Wall Press 1984.
— ed. Cadogan, George. *Jamaican Nightingale: Wonderful Adventures of Mary Seacole in Many Lands*, Stratford ON: Williams-Wallace 1987.
— *Wonderful Adventures of Mrs. Seacole in Many Lands*, ed. W.J.S. Oxford: Oxford University Press 1988. Introduction by William L. Andrews.
— ed. Salih, Sara. *Wonderful Adventures of Mrs Seacole in Many Lands*, Penguin 20th Century Classics reprint 2005.
— ed. Washington, Harriet. *Wonderful Adventures of Mrs Seacole in Many Lands*, Kaplan Publishing 2009.

Translations

Mary Seacole's Avonturen in de West en in de Krim Rotterdam: 1857.
— *Mary Seacole's Avonturen in de West en in de Krim*, With W.H. Russell voorede. Nijmegen: Ingraal 2007. New ed.

Aventures et voyages d'une Créole à Panama et en Crimée, trans., Victorine Rilliet de Constant Massé. Lausanne: Delafontaine 1858.
— *Aventures et voyages d'une Créole, Mme Seacole, Panama et en Crimée*, trans., Victorine Rilliet de Constant Massé. Nabu Press 2011 reprint.

Sources from the Nineteenth and Early Twentieth Centuries

Alexander, James Edward. *Life of a Soldier: Or, Military Service in the East and West, 2 vol.* London: Hurst & Blackett 1857.

Allan, William. *Crimean Letters: From the 41st (the Welch) Regiment 1854–56*, ed. Alister Williams. Wrexham: Bridge Books 2011.

Arnold, Robert Arthur. *From the Levant, the Black Sea, and the Danube, 2 vols.* London: Chapman & Hall 1868.

Ashley, Evelyn. *The Life and Correspondence of Henry John Temple Viscount Palmerston, 2 vols.* London: R. Bentley 1879.

Astley, John Dugdale. *Fifty Years of my Life in the World of Sport*, 4th ed. 1 vol. London: Hurst & Blackett 1895 [1894].

Blackwood, Alicia. *A Narrative of Personal Experiences & Impressions During a Residence on the Bosphorus throughout the Crimean War*, London: Hatchard 1881.

Bonham-Carter, Victor, ed., assisted by Monica Lawson. *Surgeon in the Crimea: The Experiences of George Lawson Recorded in Letters to his Family 1854–55*, London: Constable 1868.

Buzzard, Thomas. *With the Turkish Army in the Crimea and Asia Minor: A Personal Narrative*, London: John Murray 1915.

Chenu, Jean-Charles. *Rapport au Conseil de Santé des Armées sur les résultats du service médico-chirurgical pendant la campagne d'Orient en 1854–56*, Paris 1865.
— *De la mortalité dans l'armée et des moyens d'économiser la vie humaine*, Paris: Hachette 1870.

Douglas, George and Ramsay, George Dalhousie, eds. *The Panmure Papers, Being a Selection from the Correspondence of Fox Maule, Second Baron Panmure, Afterwards Eleventh Earl of Dalhousie*, KT, GCB 2 vols. London: Hodder & Stoughton 1908.

Duberly, Frances Isabella. *Mrs Duberly's War: Journal and Letters from the Crimea 1854–6*, ed. Christine Kelly. Oxford: Oxford University Press 2007.

— Duberly, Mrs Henry. *Journal Kept During the Russian War from the Departure of the Army from England in April 1854 to the Fall of Sebastopol*, London: Longman, Brown 1856.

Eyre-Todd, George, ed. *The Autobiography of William Simpson*, R.I. London: T. Fisher Unwin 1903.

Goldie, Sue M., ed. *'I have Done my Duty': Florence Nightingale in the Crimean War 1854–1856*, Manchester: Manchester University Press 1987.

Hall, John. *Observations on the Report of the Sanitary Commissioners in the Crimea, During the Years 1855 and 1856*, London: W. Clowes & Sons [1857].

Hamley, E. Bruce. *The Story of the Campaign of Sebastopol, Written in the Camp*, Edinburgh: William Blackwood & Sons 1855.

Hamlin, Cyrus. *My Life and Times.* 2nd Ed. Boston: Congregational Sunday School & Publishing Society1893.

Hume, John Richard. *Reminiscences of the Crimean Campaign with the 55th Regiment*, London: Unwin 1894.

Kelly, Mrs Tom and Stother, Samuel Kelson. From the Fleet in the Fifties: A History of the Crimean War, London: Hurst & Blackett 1902.

Kinglake, Alexander William. *The Invasion of the Crimea: Its Origin and an Account of its Progress down to the Death of Lord Raglan*, Edinburgh: Wm Blackwood & Sons 1901.

Le Fort, Léon. *Oeuvres de Léon Le Fort,* 3 vols. Paris: Félix Alcan 1895.

Luddy, Maria, ed. *The Crimean Journals of the Sisters of Mercy 1854–56*, Dublin: Four Courts 2004.

Marsh, Catherine. *Memorials of Captain Hedley Vicars*, London: James Nisbet 1856.

Mawson, Michael Hargreave, ed. *Eyewitness in the Crimea: the Crimean War Letters (1854–1856) of Lt Col George Frederick Dallas, Sometime Captain 46th Foot and ADC to Sir Robert Garrett*, London: Greenhill Books 2001.

McDonald, Lynn, ed. *Florence Nightingale: An Introduction to her Life and Family*, Waterloo ON: Wilfrid Laurier University Press 2001.
— *Florence Nightingale: The Nightingale School*, Waterloo ON: Wilfrid Laurier University Press 2009.
— *Florence Nightingale: The Crimean War*, Waterloo ON: Wilfrid Laurier University Press 2010.
— *Florence Nightingale on Wars and the War Office*, Waterloo ON: Wilfrid Laurier University Press 2011.
— *Florence Nightingale and Hospital Reform*, Waterloo ON: Wilfrid Laurier University Press 2012.

McIlraith, John. *The Life of Sir John Richardson*, London: Longmans, Green 1868.

Nightingale, Florence. *Notes on Matters Affecting the Health, Efficiency and Hospital Administration of the British Army*, London: Harrison 1858.
—*Suggestions for Thought to Searchers after Religious Truth*. 3 vols. London: Eyre & Spottiswoode 1860.
—*Notes on Hospitals*. 3rd ed. London: Longman, Green 1863.

Osborne, S.G. *Scutari and Its Hospitals*, London: Dickinson Brothers 1855.

Paget, George. *The Light Cavalry Brigade of the Crimea: Extracts from the Letters and Journal of the late Gen. Lord George Paget, KCB, during the Crimean War*, London: John Murray 1881.
Porter, Whitworth. *Life in the Trenches*, London: Longman, Brown 1856.

Ranken, George. *Six Months at Sebastopol, Being Selections from the Journal and Correspondence of the Late Major George Ranken, Royal Engineers*, ed. W. Bayne Ranken. London: Charles Westerton 1857.

Reid, Douglas Arthur. *Memories of the Crimean War January 1855 to June 1856*, London: St Catherine Press 1911.
— *Soldier-Surgeon: The Crimean War Letters of Dr Douglas A. Reid 1855–1856*, ed., Joseph O. Baylen and Alan Conway. Knoxville: University of Tennessee 1968.

Robins, Colin, annot. *The Murder of a Regiment: Winter Sketches from the Crimea 1854–1855*, Bowdong, Cheshire: Withycut House 1994.
— ed. *Captain Dunscombe's Diary: The Real Crimean War That the British Infantry Knew*, Bowdong, Cheshire: Withycut House 2003.

Robinson, Frederick. *Diary of the Crimean War*, London: Richard Bentley 1856.

Russell, William Howard. *The War: From the Landing at Gallipoli to the Death of Lord Raglan*, London: Routledge 1855.
— *The War: From the Death of Lord Raglan to the Evacuation of the Crimea*, London: Routledge 1856.
— *The Great War with Russia: The Invasion of the Crimea*, London: Routledge 1895.
— *Despatches from the Crimea*, ed. Nicolas Bentley. London: Deutsch 1906.
— *Russell's Despatches from the Crimea 1854–1856*, London: Deutsch 1966.
— *The Noise of Drums and Trumpets: W.H. Russell Reports from the Crimea,* ed. Elizabeth Grey. London: Longman 1971.
— *Russell of The Times: War Despatches and Diaries*, ed. Caroline Chapman. London: Bell & Hyman 1984.

Skene, James Henry. *With Lord Stratford in the Crimean War*, London: Richard Bentley & Son 1883.

Smith, Andrew. *Medical and Surgical History of the British Army which served in Turkey and the Crimea*. 2 vols. London: Harrison 1858.

Soyer, Alexis. *Soyer's Culinary Campaign, Being Historical Reminiscences of the Late War*, London: G. Routledge 1857.

Sullivan, Mary C., ed. *The Friendship of Florence Nightingale and Mary Clare Moore*, Philadelphia: University of Pennsylvania Press 1999.

Sutherland, John. *Report of The Sanitary Commission Dispatched to the Seat of War in the East 1855–56*, London: Harrison & Sons 1857.

Tolstoy, Leo. *Sebastopol Sketches*, trans. David McDuff. Harmondsworth: Penguin 1986 [1855].

Trollope, Anthony. *The West Indies and the Spanish Main*, London: Frank Cass 1868.

UK. *Report upon the State of the Hospitals of the British Army in the Crimea and Scutari*, London: Eyre & Spottiswoode 1855 (Parliamentary Papers 1854–5 XXXIII).
— *Report of the Commission of Inquiry into the Supplies of the British Army in the Crimea*, London: Harrison & Sons 1855.
— *Report of the Commissioners appointed to Inquire into the Regulations affecting the Sanitary Condition of the Army and the Treatment of the Sick and Wounded*, London: HMSO 1858.

Vieth, Frederick Harris Dawes. *Recollections of the Crimean Campaign and the Expedition to Kinburn in 1855*, Montreal: John Lovell 1907.

Wood, Evelyn. *The Crimea in 1854 and 1894*, London: Chapman & Hall 1895.

Secondary Sources — Print

Akinsanya, Justus A. *An African 'Florence Nightingale': A Biography of Chief (Dr) Mrs Kofoworola Abeni Pratt*, Ibadan: Vantage 1987.

Anionwu, Elizabeth N. *A Short History of Mary Seacole: A Resource for Nurses and Students*, Royal College of Nursing 2005.

Atkins, John Black. *The Life of Sir William Howard Russell, the First Special Correspondent*, 2 vols. London: John Murray 1911.

Barnham, Kay. *Florence Nightingale: The Lady of the Lamp*, Lewes: White-Thomson 2002.

Battiscombe, Georgina. *Shaftesbury: A Biography of the Seventh Earl 1801–1885*, London: Constable 1974.

Bostridge, Mark. *Florence Nightingale: The Woman and her Legend*, London: Viking 2008.

Buss, Julia. *Black Nightingale: Mary Seacole, Hero of the Crimean War*, San Francisco: David Millett Publications 2011.

Calder, Angus. *Gods, Mongrels and Demons*, London: Bloomsbury 2004.

Carnegie, M. Elizabeth. *The Path We Tread: Blacks in Nursing*, 3rd ed. Sudbury MA: Jones & Bartlett 2000 [1995].

Castor, Harriet. *Mary Seacole*, New York/London: Franklin Watts 1999.

Cherry, Barbara and Jacob, Susan R. *Contemporary Nursing: Issues, Trends and Management*, St Louis: Mosby 1999.

Collicott, Sylvia L. *The Story of Mary Seacole*, London: Macmillan Education 2001.

Compton, Piers. *Colonel's Lady and Camp Follower: The Story of Women in the Crimean War*. London: Robert Hale 1970.

Cook, Edward T. The Life of Florence Nightingale, 2 vols. London: Macmillan 1913.

Cottone, Gregory R., ed. *Disaster Medicine*, Philadelphia: Elsevier Mosby 2006.

Donald, Graeme. *Loose Cannons: 101 Myths, Mishaps and Misadventurers of Military History*, Oxford: Osprey 2009.

Figes, Orlando. *Crimea: The Last Crusade*, London: Allen Lane 2010.

Fish, Cheryl J. 'Travelling Medicine Chest: Mary Seacole "Plays Doctor" at Colonial Crossroads in Panama and in the Crimea,' *Black and White Women's Travel Narratives*, Gainesville FL: University Press of Florida 2004 65–95.

Fryer, Peter. 'Mary Seacole.' *Staying Power: The History of Black People in Britain*, London: Pluto 1984.

Furneaux, Rupert. *The First War Correspondent: William Howard Russell of The Times*, London: Cassell 1944.

Gardiner, Juliet, ed. *'Seacole, Mary,' Who's Who in British History*, London: Collins & Brown 2000.

Hankinson, Alan. *Man of Wars: William Howard Russell of The Times*, London: Heinemann 1982.

Harrison, Paul. *Who Was Mary Seacole?* London: Wayland 2007.

Hart, Ellen. *Man Born to Live: Life and Work of Henry Dunant, Founder of the Red Cross*, London: Victor Gollancz 1953.

Hewitt, Hermi Hyacinth. *Trailblazers in Nursing Education: A Caribbean Perspective, 1946–1986*, Kingston Jamaica: Canoe Press 2002.

Hibbert, Christopher. *The Destruction of Lord Raglan: A Tragedy of the Crimean War*, London: Longmans 1961.

Huntley, Eric L. *Two Lives: Florence Nightingale and Mary Seacole*, London: Bogle-L'Ouverture 1993.

Johnson, Boris. 'Florence Nightingale and Mary Seacole: Who Pioneered Nursing,' *Johnson's Life of London: The People Who Made the City That Made the World*, London: Harper 2011 282–307

Klainberg, Marilyn. *An Historical Overview of Nursing*, Sudbury Mass: Jones & Bartlett 2009.

Lambert, David and Lester, Alan, eds. *Colonial Lives Across the British Empire: Imperial Careering in the Long Nineteenth Century*, Cambridge: Cambridge University Press 2006.

Lynch, Emma. *The Life of Mary Seacole*, Oxford: Heinemann 2006.

Mayo, John Horsley. *Medals and Decorations of the British Army and Navy*, London: Archibald Constable 1897. Vol. 2 Crimea 1854–6.

McAllister, Margaret and John B. Lowe. *The Resilient Nurse: Empowering Your Practice*, New York: Springer 2011.

McDonald, Lynn. *Florence Nightingale at First Hand*, London: Continuum 2010.
— 'Nightingale and Seacole: Nursing's Bitter Rivalry,' *History Today* 62,9 (September 2012):10–16.
— 'Florence Nightingale and Mary Seacole on Nursing and Health Care,' *Journal of Advanced Nursing* 2013.
— 'Wonderful Adventures — How did Mary Seacole come to be Viewed as a Pioneer of Modern Nursing?' *The Times Literary Supplement* (6 December 2013):14–15.
— 'Florence Nightingale and Mary Seacole: Which is the Forgotten Hero of Health Care and Why,' *Scottish Medical Journal* 59,1 (1 February 2014):66–69.

McLoughlin, Kate. *Authoring War: The Literary Representation of War from the Iliad*, Cambridge: Cambridge University Press 2011.

McMahon, Deirdre H. "'My Own Dear Sons': Discursive Maternity and Proper British Bodies in Wonderful Adventures of Mrs Seacole in Many Lands,' Rosenman, Ellen Bayuk and Klaver, Claudia C., eds. *Other Mothers: Beyond the Maternal Ideal*, Columbus: Ohio State University Press 2008 181–201.

Mitra, S.M. *The Life and Letters of Sir John Hall MD, KCB, FRCS*, London: Longmans, Green 1911.

Moorcroft, Christine and Magnusson, Magnus. *Mary Seacole 1805–1881*, London: Channel Four Learning 2002 [2000].

Moore, Henry Charles. *Noble Deeds of the World's Heroines*, London: Religious Tract Society 1903 (Online 2009).

Morris, Helen. *Portrait of a Chef: The Life of Alexis Soyer*, New York: Macmillan 1938.

Page, Yolanda Williams, ed. *Encyclopedia of African American Women Writers*, 2 vols. Westport CT: Greenwood 2007.

Peck, John. *War, the Army and Victorian Literature*, Houndmills, Hants: Macmillan 1998.

Pemberton, W. Baring. *Battles of the Crimean War*, London: B.T. Batsford 1962.

Ponting, Clive. *The Crimean War: The Truth behind the Myth*, London: Chatto & Windus 2004.

Ramdin, Ron. *Mary Seacole*, London: Haus 2005.

Rappaport, Helen. 'Seacole, Mary (1805–1881) Jamaica,' *An Encyclopedia of Women Social Reformers*, Santa Barbara CA: ABC-Clio 2001 2:631–33.

Robinson, Jane. *Mary Seacole: The Charismatic Black Nurse Who Became a Heroine of the Crimea*, London: Constable 2005.

Royle, Trevor. Crimea: The Great Crimean War 1854–1856, New York: St Martin's Press 2000 [1999].

Rushdie, Salman. *Grimus: a Novel*, New York: Overlook Press 1979 [1975].
— *The Satanic Verses*, New York: Viking 1988.

Schama, Simon. *A History of Britain*. New York: Hyperion 2002.

Shepherd, John. *The Crimean Doctors: A History of the British Medical Services in the Crimean War*, 2 vols. Liverpool: Liverpool University Press 1991.

Singh, Simon and Edzard, Ernst. *Trick or Treatment: Alternative Medicine on Trial*, London: Corgi Bantam 2008.

Silver, Christopher. *Renkioi: Brunel's Forgotten Crimean War Hospital*, Sevenoaks: Valonia 2007.

Small, Hugh. *Florence Nightingale: Avenging Angel*, London: Constable 1998.

Smith, Fred. *A Short History of the Royal Army Medical Corps*, Aldershot: Gale & Polden 1929.

Stevenhoved, Susanne. *Six Hundred Women and One Man: Nurses on Stamps*, Kolding: Danish Museum of Nursing History 2004.

Williams, Brian. *The Life and World of Mary Seacole*, Oxford: Heinemann 2003.

Wilson, A.N. *The Victorians*, London: Arrow 2002.

BBC

BBC Learning Zone. 'The Work of Florence Nightingale and Mary Seacole' (drama). Classic Clips 5.44 clip 13650 2012.

BBC History. 'Mary Seacole (1805–1881)' website, 2012.

BBC Famous People. 'Mary Seacole Famous Nurse.'

BBC Knowledge. 'Mary Seacole: A Hidden History,' September 2000 for Black History Season, rebroadcast by BBC2 in 2005.

BBC School Radio. 'History — the Victorians.'

BBC. 'Horrible Histories: Mary Seacole' and 'Florence Nightingale and Mary Seacole.'

Miscellaneous Films and Electronic Sources

Caribbean Icons in Science, Technology & Innovation. 'A Caribbean Florence Nightingale: Mary Seacole, Nurse,' Trinidad: National Institute of Higher Education, Research, Science and Technology.

Channel 4. 'Mary Seacole: The Real Angel of the Crimea,' 2005. Available online.

Dabydeen, David; Gilmore, John; Jones, Cecily, eds. *Oxford Companion to Black British History,* Online source.

Seaton, Helen J. 'Another Florence Nightingale? The Rediscovery of Mary Seacole,' The Victorian Web online.

Young Foundation. *Social Silicon Valleys: A Manifesto for Social Innovation,* Spring 2006 online.

Index

Iguana Books

iguanabooks.com

If you enjoyed *Mary Seacole: The Making of the Myth*...
Look for other books coming soon from Iguana Books! Subscribe to our blog for updates as they happen.

iguanabooks.com/blog/

If you're a writer ...
Iguana Books is always looking for great new writers, in every genre. We produce primarily ebooks but, as you can see, we do the occasional print book as well. Visit us at iguanabooks.com to see what Iguana Books has to offer both emerging and established authors.

iguanabooks.com/publishing-with-iguana/

If you're looking for another good book ...
All Iguana Books books are available on our website. We pride ourselves on making sure that every Iguana book is a great read.

iguanabooks.com/bookstore/

Visit our bookstore today and support your favourite author.

IGUANA

Lightning Source UK Ltd.
Milton Keynes UK
UKOW03f0625260914

239162UK00003B/86/P